WAYNE FROGGATT

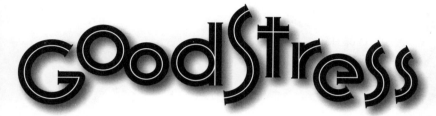

THE LIFE THAT CAN BE YOURS

HarperCollins*Publishers New Zealand*

By the same author
CHOOSE TO BE HAPPY
Your step-by-step guide

First published 1997

HarperCollins*Publishers (New Zealand) Limited*
P.O. Box 1, Auckland

ISBN 1 86950 256 6

Designed by Pages Literary Pursuits
Back cover photo by Heather Froggatt
Printed by GP Print Ltd, Wellington, New Zealand

Contents

Contents

Part Two: The Foundations for Effective Stress Management

Part Three: Building on the Foundations — Practical Skills for Coping with Life

Contents

Acknowledgements

As with my previous book, *Choose to be Happy*, many of the contributors to *GoodStress* will remain anonymous — the clients who have used the methods described in the following pages and, over the years, have provided me with feedback which has helped me refine them.

I also owe a debt of gratitude to colleagues who have assisted me. I am especially grateful to David Ramsden and Sonya Mason, who have offered encouragement and suggestions from the early stages of the project and, along with Julie Parkinson, have reviewed the book in its entirety.

Other colleagues have contributed invaluable guidance, assessment and comment on specific topics relating to their specialist areas of expertise: Dr Paul Hendy, Jenni McKinley, Dr Ruth Williams, Cathi Pharazyn and Greta Wham.

My family once again deserve special recognition for their patience while I disappeared to write this book, and forbearance with my constant requests to provide a lay person's point of view on various aspects of it.

This book, like the last, is solidly based on the principles of Rational Emotive Behaviour Therapy and Cognitive Therapy. Consequently, I acknowledge an ongoing debt to Drs Albert Ellis and Aaron Beck. To these I add a third innovator — Dr Dominic DiMattia, who has developed these principles for use in the workplace and in general stress management. The originator of Rational Effectiveness Training, he has graciously provided *GoodStress* with its foreword, and I hope the book will prove a worthy addition to the growing literature on RET.

Wayne Froggatt
1997

Dr DiMattia, for some years Associate Executive Director of the Institute for Rational-Emotive Therapy in New York, is the originator of Rational Effectiveness Training. He is currently Vice President of Human Resources for Café Concepts, New York.

Foreword

It would be an understatement to say that conditions around the world are changing very rapidly. We are all aware of the enormous changes in both our personal and work environments which have taken place during the past twenty-five years.

Although change is exciting, it can also produce many conditions which are difficult to cope with effectively. The cybernetic revolution has created an information explosion which, at times, seems impossible to keep up with. International travel has brought different cultures into collision with each other. The family and local community no longer regulate our values and behaviour. Conflicting influences from around the world often leave individuals helpless over deciding how to manage their lives. It is becoming increasingly difficult to arrange our lives in such a manner as to avoid stressful conditions.

The only solution, therefore, is to learn to handle these stressors in a productive and satisfying way. *GoodStress: The life that can be yours* clearly points out the distinction between harmful and motivating stress, and presents many tools to alleviate the effects of unpleasant events in our lives.

Without some external pressures, life becomes boring and meaningless, but it is important we recognise when these pressures are taking a toll on our bodies and quality of life. The comprehensive and clear treatment of external pressure offered by this book can help us all as long as we commit ourselves to a life-long self-management programme. Our bodies respond better when we exercise; in the same manner, our minds respond better when we practise the Rational Effectiveness techniques which have been developed from the pioneering work of Dr Albert Ellis. Learning to recognise and then challenge our demanding thoughts and philosophies can lead to a very satisfying and productive life.

If you constantly follow the recommendations in this book, your body and mind will be more energised than you could believe possible.

Good luck on your journey to a satisfying and healthy life.

Dominic J. DiMattia, EdD

Part One

Understanding and Diagnosing Your Stress

1
What is Stress?

Stress has got a bad name. People dislike it. Most view it as something to avoid at any cost. Many people abuse alcohol or drugs to medicate their bad feelings, some use violence to control their circumstances, others act unassertively to avoid the discomfort of disapproval — all solutions that create new problems of their own.

A whole industry has grown up to help people deal with stress. *Stress management* has become a hot topic for self-help books and training seminars. Unfortunately, many of the books and expensive seminars make grand promises they do not fulfil, leaving people disillusioned.

Why are stress-management programmes often ineffective — and many solutions worse than the problem? The main reason is this: contrary to what most people think, stress itself is not the problem! To understand why, let's begin with a brief introduction to the nature of stress and its causes.

Introducing stress

What is this phenomenon people are so eager to avoid? Here we run into a complication. When we talk about stress, we can mean two different things. We may be referring to things *outside* us — aspects of our circumstances or surroundings we regard as stressful. Or we may be talking about what is going on *inside* — what we are feeling. Just what does the word mean?

Until this century, *stress* was a synonym for *hardship*, *adversity* or *affliction*. So, in its older sense, it referred to *influences on* a person.

About fifty years ago a young doctor named Hans Selye began using the word *stress* to describe the body's *responses* to influences such as viruses, extreme temperatures and emotional states like anger or fear. Selye saw these responses as the body's way of *adapting* to external influences. His use of the word to include both influences and responses has since entered common usage. Stress is now seen as a process in which the body fights back or attempts to adapt to external influences or challenges.

In its modern sense, therefore, the word *stress* refers to both (1) an *event* or circumstance (the stress trigger or stressor) which we perceive to be a challenge, and (2) a set of *symptoms* — physical, emotional and behavioural (the stress reaction) — which occur when our entire system gears up to deal with the event.

Events and circumstances include both *external* events — such as a car accident or losing your job — and *internal* events — like feeling excited or the heart skipping a beat (we often react to things that happen inside us, as well as outside). Symptoms include such things as the heart beating more rapidly, faster breathing or excessive sweating.

Why do human beings feel stress?

Stress occurs when your view of an event upsets your balance and puts pressure on you to adjust. What goes on in the mind affects the body. The brain sends signals through the nervous system, telling glands to secrete chemicals and muscles to tighten.

All sorts of things can act as stressors, including happy events, such as having a baby. A lack of stimulating events can also be a stressor, by producing the unpleasant need to adjust to boredom. A single event may not be a stressor, but a number of events occurring together can be. Whatever the source, stress occurs when there is a strain on your coping resources.

Where does the stress response originate from?

The stress response is a carry-over from the days when humans were regularly exposed to physical dangers like wild animals, other hostile humans and food shortages. What we call the fight–flight response — in which adrenalin is secreted, blood flow to the muscles increases and breathing speeds up — is designed to prepare the body for physical action. Unfortunately, in modern life this arousal happens mostly in situations that don't call for physical action. Consequently, you are left with your body 'all tensed up with nowhere to go'.

Nature and nurture are both involved. There may be, as we shall see later, some inherited predispositions, but these are overlaid by learning throughout life.

The stages of stress

There are three main ways to react to a stressor. Avoidance (the *flight* response), resistance (the *fight* response) or adaptation (the *accommodate* response). Each of these reactions can be functional or dysfunctional, depending on the situation. Note that nature does not always know best here. Our bodies, unfortunately, often gear up for physical action when it is not required. To have your muscles tighten, heart speed up and breathing rate increase may be useful if someone is coming at you with a knife, but it is less helpful when someone makes a critical comment in a committee meeting.

Your body (and mind) has only so much ability to cope with stress. According to Selye, people usually go through three stages when reacting to a stress trigger.[1]

The first stage is *alarm* — surprise and anxiety because of inexperience at dealing with a new situation.

The second stage involves either *avoidance*, *resistance* or *adaptation*. Either you remove yourself from the situation, or you begin trying to cope with it (by resisting or adapting), and continue for as long as it takes to deal with it (or as long as your system can manage).

The third and final stage is *exhaustion*. This occurs when you keep reacting long enough for the system's resources to become depleted.

It is possible to move through these stages and cope without becoming too exhausted; but, unfortunately, it is all too easy to end up stuck in one of them.

A high level of physical and emotional arousal that lasts too long is unhelpful. If you are extremely angry, for instance, you aren't able to think clearly. The unpleasant physical symptoms, if they continued long enough, might damage your body.

Why some people have more trouble with stress

We all react differently to a perceived challenge. Some people get sick or depressed, become violent, withdraw or abuse substances. Others can laugh off problems or take them as they come. Why is this?

How we react depends on how we *perceive* our ability to cope with a particular challenge, and how we *evaluate* our ability to manage. For instance, I may perceive that I can cope moderately well and evaluate this as acceptable, and so feel only moderately stressed. Someone else may likewise perceive they can cope moderately well, but — because they think they should be able to cope 'perfectly' — they evaluate this as unacceptable, thus becoming highly stressed. Our beliefs — that is, our perceptions and evaluations — play a crucial role in stress management, and it is in this respect that people differ so much.

Some people are predisposed to have more trouble with stress than others. A person's predisposition, as we shall see later, may be both genetically inherited and learned.

The most significant predisposition lies in beliefs and attitudes. Stress triggers are not distressing unless we perceive them as such. There is only a limited number of physical sensations we can experience, and our body reacts to all stress triggers in much the same way — increased heart rate, respiration and blood pressure. There are, however, a great many ways in which these sensations can be perceived and evaluated. We learn to put different values on different stress triggers, some positive and some negative.

Is stress always a bad thing?

Earlier I suggested that stress itself is not a problem. This may sound strange at first; however, some stress is essential to your survival and happiness. You need it to motivate you and keep you alert. Even when asleep you are slightly stressed. In fact, without some degree of stress you would be dead.

Understimulation leads to boredom and sometimes depression. Many people actually seek to increase their stress by deliberately jumping out of aeroplanes or engaging in other high-risk activities. The question is not whether stress is good or bad in itself, but rather how much, at what times and under what conditions it is helpful or unhelpful. Helpful stress we will call *goodstress*, and its dysfunctional opposite *distress*.

Goodstress

Goodstress involves physical sensations, emotions and behaviours that are (1) moderate rather than extreme, (2) help you solve your problems and cope with life effectively, and (3) reduce when they are no longer needed.

Goodstress occurs when you either:

1. perceive that you have the capabilities required to deal with a situation; or
2. perceive that you lack the capability but evaluate this deficiency in a rational way. You might, for example, view lack of success in some area as sad or disappointing, but not as proof you are a total failure as a human being.

The mild anxiety that enhances performance, the sensation of being in love and the adrenalin high of exciting activities are examples of goodstress. Goodstress also includes negative emotional states like concern, irritation, annoyance or disappointment. While these are unpleasant feelings, they are not disabling and, if handled appropriately, they can motivate productive action.

Distress

Distress, in contrast, involves (1) extreme levels of emotional upset, dysfunctional behaviour and physical complications, ranging from the high anxiety of panic to the depths of depression, that (2) hinder you from coping effectively with your problems, and (3) carry on beyond the point where they are useful.

Distress occurs when you perceive that you lack the capabilities required to meet the demands of a situation *and* evaluate this deficiency in two or three self-defeating ways:

1. You see it as catastrophic or intolerable.
2. You think it shouldn't be happening to you.
3. You believe it proves something bad about you as a person.

Distress may occur through being obsessively in love, getting so anxious it impairs performance, letting irritation escalate into hostile anger, and the like.

Distress is sometimes complicated by what we call a *secondary problem* — having a problem about having a problem. Downing yourself or feeling guilty because you are stressed are examples of secondary problems.

How much stress is good or bad?

How much stress is 'good' and how much is 'bad' varies from person to person. Some people are happy to live a passive life, which others would find boring. Others are only happy when they strive to excel or are stretched in various directions. Most are happiest in between these two extremes. Generally, we dislike both a total lack of stress and an excess of it.

A complete definition of stress

We can summarise the above into a concise but informative definition of stress, one that we will use throughout the book.

Stress refers to:

1. an event or circumstance (the stress *trigger* or *stressor*) which you perceive to be a challenge; and

2. a set of symptoms — physical, emotional and behavioural (the stress *reaction*) — which occur when your entire system gears up to deal with the trigger.

A stress *reaction* can be:

1. *Dysfunctional*, i.e. the symptoms are excessive, hinder coping and persist. *Dis*tress occurs when you perceive that you lack the capabilities required to meet the demands of a situation, and you evaluate this deficiency in a self-defeating way, perhaps creating a secondary problem out of the original stress.
2. *Functional*, i.e. the symptoms are moderate, help you cope and diminish within a reasonable time. *Good*stress occurs when you perceive either that you have the capabilities required to deal with a situation, or that you lack the capability but evaluate this deficiency in a rational way.

Improving your own stress management

Shortly we will learn how to strengthen attitudes that contribute to good stress management. First, though, let us note that human beings seem to have some built-in drives that motivate them to strive at coping with life. As Hans Selye has pointed out, 'the aim of life is to continue its existence'.[2]

We want to do more than just survive, though. Most people want to feel good and avoid discomfort. We want to maximise our pleasure and minimise our pain. When we talk about stress management, are we not talking about handling life in ways that leave us feeling good — and help us avoid feeling bad?

The big question is: How well do we do this? Chances are, your answer will be: 'Not as well as I'd like to!' The desire to improve oneself and one's circumstances is a basic part of human nature. Unfortunately, as we shall see, another part of our human inheritance is to go about this in ineffective and inefficient ways. That is why most people need to learn how to manage stress. Showing you how you can do this is the purpose of this book.

How to use this book

Let us take an advance look at what lies ahead, and see how you can use this book most efficiently to achieve your goal of effective stress management.

Part One will help you understand what stress is, how to recognise its signs and symptoms, what triggers it, and its underlying causes. You will probably want to read this part only once, to gain a general understanding of stress and its origins.

Part Two looks at how you can manage stress. This section of the book is very important. It explores the prerequisites, or essential requirements, for effective stress management, providing a firm underpinning of basic principles on which the remainder of the book can build.

Part Three applies these principles through a number of practical strategies for dealing with stress. This is also an important section. Not all the practical strategies covered will be useful to you, and of those that are, some will be more helpful than others. Accordingly, you may wish to pick out the chapters that are most relevant and concentrate on those. The section closes with a demonstration of how all of the learning can be applied to a specific area of life — the workplace.

If you would like to explore any aspect of stress and its management in more detail, at the end of most chapters you will find suggestions for further reading. If you have access to the Internet, at the end of the book is a selection of sites on the Worldwide Web where you can find free information relevant to most of the chapters. This is followed by a listing of professional books and articles on various aspects of stress management.

To summarise: Part One may need reading once only. Read and study Part Two carefully. Part Three may be read selectively, according to the areas that are problematic for you. I wish you all the best as you begin your journey from distress to goodstress!

2
Recognising Your Symptoms

One of the first steps to avoiding stress is to recognise the signs at an early stage. Accordingly, this chapter will list the symptoms of general stress (or, more particularly, *distress*) and describe some related conditions that may require professional help.

The general signs of stress

Tick the symptoms under each heading that you identify as applying to you.

Specific physical symptoms

Stress can show in many physical symptoms. The most common are listed here:

- ☐ Restlessness
- ☐ Excitability, over alertness, keyed up, easily startled
- ☐ Increased heart rate and blood pressure
- ☐ Irritability
- ☐ Shortness of breath, faster breathing
- ☐ Muscle tension, especially in neck or lower back
- ☐ Headaches
- ☐ Poor sleep
- ☐ Fatigue, low energy
- ☐ Pain
- ☐ Dry mouth/throat, flushed, hot face, sweating
- ☐ Weakness, dizziness
- ☐ Trembling, nervous tics, grinding of teeth
- ☐ Frequent need to pass water
- ☐ Diarrhoea or constipation
- ☐ Indigestion, queasiness in stomach, vomiting
- ☐ Loss of appetite, or eating more
- ☐ Other physical symptoms: _____

General health problems

Stress is often associated with an increased likelihood of physical health problems:

- ☐ Digestion problems
- ☐ Increased susceptibility to colds and influenza
- ☐ High blood pressure, strokes, angina, heart attacks
- ☐ Migraine, chronic pain
- ☐ Stomach and duodenal ulcers, ulcerative colitis
- ☐ Irritable bowel syndrome
- ☐ Miscellaneous health problems, including diabetes, rheumatoid arthritis, allergies, cancer, asthma, baldness, eczema
- ☐ Other health problems: _____

Emotional and cognitive changes

Emotional and cognitive changes associated with stress commonly include:

- ☐ Anxiety, worrying
- ☐ Difficulty concentrating, wandering thoughts
- ☐ Forgetfulness
- ☐ Moodiness, depression
- ☐ Loss of interest, dissatisfaction with life or job
- ☐ Self-downing
- ☐ Hostile anger
- ☐ Other emotions (e.g. guilt, loss of enjoyment, highly changeable emotional state): _____

Behaviours

Some behavioural changes are often associated with stress:

- ☐ Impatience, impulsiveness, hyperactivity
- ☐ Short temper, aggressiveness, abuse of partner and/or children
- ☐ Accident proneness
- ☐ Urge to cry, run or hide, isolation/withdrawal
- ☐ Smoking more
- ☐ Use of prescription drugs, especially tranquillisers
- ☐ Alcohol abuse
- ☐ Illegal drug use

- ☐ High-pitched, nervous laughter
- ☐ Poor motivation, poor performance, procrastination, absenteeism
- ☐ Uncooperativeness, rebelliousness
- ☐ Workaholic behaviour — would rather keep busy than sleep, unhappy when activity stops
- ☐ Other behaviours: _____

Concerns expressed by others

Finally, stress may be indicated when other people begin to express concern:

- ☐ Partner or children complain that you are absent, preoccupied or grouchy much of the time
- ☐ At work people comment that you are making more mistakes or forgetting things
- ☐ People remark that your sporting performance has declined
- ☐ Other concerns: _____

Burnout

There is an extreme stress condition called burnout, which, although it may occur under many circumstances, is commonly associated with the workplace. See page 229 for a description.

Clinical stress conditions

There are a few conditions that go beyond generalised stress and are regarded as diagnosable mental-health disorders.[1] These may warrant professional intervention.

Post-traumatic stress disorder (PTSD)

PTSD may occur following exposure to an unusually traumatic event involving actual or threatened death or serious injury, coupled with intense feelings of fear, horror or helplessness.

The person affected keeps reliving the event through intrusive and distressing thoughts, images, dreams, flashbacks, hallucinations, illusions or marked distress when reminded of the event. They try to avoid anything that reminds them — feelings, thoughts, conversations, activities, places or people. They may 'forget' aspects of the event or detach from other people. They exhibit symptoms of hyperarousal — such as insomnia, angry outbursts, irritability, poor concentration, excessive vigilance, increased startle response — that were not present prior to the event.

Symptoms may occur either immediately or at a later stage, and they last longer than one month.

Acute stress disorder

Acute stress disorder has characteristics similar to those of PTSD, except that they appear within four weeks of the trauma and last from two days to four weeks.

Adjustment disorder

Adjustment disorder involves a response (distress, or impairment of job, academic or social functioning) to an identifiable stress trigger which is excessive for the degree of stress involved. It occurs within three months of the event and lasts no longer than six months. Unlike post-traumatic stress disorder and acute stress disorder, the reaction is regarded as being out of proportion to whatever triggered it.

Other related clinical conditions

There are a few other mental-health conditions which may be related to stress. Because they are relatively common but require different treatment from general stress, it is important to be able to recognise them.

Generalised anxiety disorder

GAD is characterised by excessive worrying about multiple concerns, coupled with symptoms such as restlessness, feeling excessively tired, poor concentration, irritability, tension and poor sleep. These symptoms occur most days for at least six months. Functioning is affected, though not always severely.

Panic disorder

A *panic attack* involves a severe fear or discomfort that peaks within ten minutes. There are strong symptoms such as chest pain, chills or hot flushes, a choking feeling, dizziness, pounding of the heart, nausea, sweating, shortness of breath, trembling, and fears of dying, losing control or going insane.

Panic disorder involves a series of panic attacks coupled with worry about having another attack. The attacks may have a recognisable trigger, though often not. Repeated panic attacks usually lead to avoidance of situations which come to be associated with them.

Major depressive episode

Depression is one of the most common disorders for which people seek help. It is characterised by (1) lowered mood, or (2) loss of interest or pleasure, or (3) both. This is coupled with at least three or four of the following:

- Appetite or weight changes
- Sleep disturbance
- Fatigue
- Increased or decreased activity levels
- Guilt
- Poor concentration
- Death wishes or suicidal ideas

These symptoms are present most of the day, most days, for at least two weeks. Functioning is usually impaired, sometimes quite severely.

Assessing your own stress

Check the clinical conditions described above. If you think any apply to you, consider seeing your doctor or another health professional for a formal assessment.

Note the general-stress symptoms you ticked at the start of the chapter. By being aware of these, you can use them as alarm signals that stress is increasing. You can then take action before matters get out of hand. As we shall see later, knowing yourself is a key step to effective stress management.

3
What Triggers Your Stress?

The causes of stress are many and varied. Knowing what you typically react to is a part of knowing yourself and will help you identify things you can watch out for and, in some cases, take action to change.

This chapter lists the common stress triggers. In the following chapter, we will examine what it is within human beings that determines how they react to those triggers.

Stress triggers

The events and circumstances that can set off a stress response are numerous. Tick any items in the following list relevant to you, and write in the space provided the specific aspects that apply. Add any unlisted items.

☐ *Family problems*
The increasing isolation of nuclear families, the lonely demands of solo parenting, marital tensions, a problem drinker, violence and difficult children can all be triggers for distress in family settings.

_____

_____

☐ *Workplace problems*
Employees may be distressed when they perceive they lack power, they have too much or too little work, there is under- or overpromotion, authority and responsibility do not match, objectives or requirements are unclear or there is conflict between multiple job demands; also when they have to contend with inadequate training, a poor physical working environment, irregular hours of work, sexual harassment or low job security.

Managers and executives have problems when they find it hard to delegate, their staff are incompetent or poorly trained, they lack control and certainty, or they are not used to the new 'participation model' and perceive they have been stripped of their power and authority.

Being in the wrong job can be distressful — when, for example, a high-energy risk-taker is in a boring, repetitive job, or a low-energy, safety-conscious person is in a high-flying job

☐ *Unemployment*

Adapting to unemployment may involve overcoming financial problems, loss of status and self-regard, and a fear of never again obtaining meaningful work.

☐ *Lifestyle changes*

Any change — even if positive — can be distressful. This may include such events as moving house, starting or finishing education, getting married, having children, divorce, taking on a new job or different type of work, promotion or retirement.

☐ *Developmental changes*

Progression through the various phases of life brings a series of stress triggers. On moving from childhood into adolescence there is pressure to conform with peers, engage in sexual activity, take drugs, perform educationally, handle conflicts with parents, develop a body image and sex-role identity, and achieve independence from parents. Middle age involves coping with adolescents, dependent elderly parents and a growing realisation that some aspirations may never be fulfilled. Old age may bring enforced retirement, lack of status, failing health and financial insecurity.

☐ *Gender-based stresses*

In the modern world, women are expected to be less emotional and more businesslike than in previous times, and men more sensitive and in touch with their emotions. Adjusting to these and other changing gender roles can result in conflict and confusion about identity.

□ *Cultural stresses*

Throughout the world, there is growing pressure for the recognition of minority groups. The stresses of adaptation to a newly bicultural society in New Zealand, for example, are mirrored in other countries, as different cultures strive to take account of each other.

□ *Discrimination*

To be picked out on the basis of race, age or sex can mean harassment and difficulty getting work or obtaining finance.

□ *Pressure to achieve status*

Stress is often triggered through internal and external demands to perform at high levels, to possess consumer items or have a fashionable appearance, or to achieve academic, material or sporting success.

□ *City life*

Increasing migration to cities means adapting to traffic, pollution, noise, crime and isolation.

□ *Rural life*

Country living can entail being at a distance from medical, education and other services, living in isolation from other people, and coping with a downturn in many rural economies with post offices and other facilities closing.

□ *Noise*

Motor vehicles, aircraft, factories, music, the telephone, television sets and stereos are all sources of noise that can create strain.

☐ *Geographical isolation*

People increasingly live away from the support of their extended families. The members of some occupational groups, such as police and bank officers, have to regularly change their social circle.

☐ *Technology*

The spread of high-tech communications means that bad news spreads rapidly. Television exposes people to incessant advertising and frequent violence, and discourages exercise of both body and brain, often resulting in boredom. Improvements in transport mean long car journeys, constant danger of accident, fear of flying, and the need to make rapid adjustments to changes in time zone, climate and culture

---

☐ *Commerce*

Planned obsolescence and high-pressure advertising are an increasing factor of modern life.

☐ *Positive events*

Even essentially happy events, such as being in love, getting married, having children, being promoted or moving to a better house can act as triggers for stress.

☐ *Internal stress triggers*

Internal events are just as likely as external events to act as stress triggers . Physical illness stresses the body, either temporarily, as with a cold or influenza, or longer term, when there is a major illness, disfigurement or disability. People may also react to passing changes in body functioning, such as the heart missing a beat or a bout of indigestion.

☐ *Other triggers*

How do external events trigger internal stress?

Stress triggers operate at more than one level. There are *major events*, such as natural disasters, accidents, war, imprisonment, divorce and bereavement. But more common are the *daily hassles* — an overload of responsibilities, arguments with one's partner, missing the bus, being criticised and so on.

One or a few challenging events, especially daily hassles, will often not be distressful; but a number that accumulate or coincide may have a significant effect. When a variety of stressors have built up, you may react to some essentially trivial event in a way that surprises both you and others — it is the straw that breaks the camel's back. As already noted, even positive events may lead to distress when too many of them occur at once.

Remember, though: *events and circumstances are not distressful unless you perceive, interpret and evaluate them as such.* What is distressful to one person may be exciting and stimulating to another. While there are major events to which most people would react with distress, there are still variations between people in the level and duration of their distress. When it comes to daily hassles, there can be an even greater variety of individual responses.

Identify your top stress triggers

List your top five stress triggers here, in order of their significance to you:

1. _____
2. _____
3. _____
4. _____
5. _____

Your personal inventory of typical stress triggers will serve some useful purposes:

- You can see if there are any patterns. Do you tend to react to particular people, or in certain situations, or when you are in certain moods? Analyse how you typically feel and behave in response to those triggers. Use your reactions as warning signs that it is time to take action.
- You can develop and rehearse appropriate coping strategies, such as assertiveness and relaxation. This will prepare you to handle the people

or situations to which you typically react, and control dysfunctional states like tension or hostility before they get out of hand.

- Finally, you can set about changing the triggers that are open to change — and accepting the ones that are not.

4
Are You Predisposed to Distress?

As we have seen, the same stressor can lead to different reactions in different people. What is it within individuals that determines how they react to external stress triggers?

Your biology

There is growing evidence that biological make-up plays a significant part in how people respond to life events.[1] Human beings appear to be born with differing temperaments, which are observable in the first month and are usually retained throughout life. Temperament is reflected in such characteristics as activity level, adaptability, physical sensitivity, intensity of reaction, the prevalence of positive or negative moods, and perseverance.[2]

High arousability

Although many aspects of temperament affect a person's reaction to stressors, one in particular is what can be called 'high arousability'. It appears that some people experience a greater sensitivity to stimuli in their environment, and their physical reactions are correspondingly more intense. It has been shown, for example, that people with a Type A personality (to be discussed shortly) exhibit enhanced adrenalin and noradrenalin secretion.[3]

High arousability shows in overreactivity, a tendency to worry, and sometimes in clinical conditions such as generalised anxiety, phobias and obsessive-compulsiveness.

Biology, learning and change

There is more to personality, though, than biochemistry. Environment is also involved.[4] A person's biological inheritance is built on through learning from the moment of birth. A biological tendency to high arousability, for example, is likely to be amplified by continued attempts to avoid uncomfortable feelings.

33

Note, too, that having a biological factor in a stress problem doesn't mean things are hopeless, simply that hard work will be needed to overcome tendencies basic to one's personality. While it is not possible with our present state of knowledge to change a person's biological make-up, it is possible to make significant changes in any faulty learning, and to develop strategies to compensate for any unhelpful aspects of one's biochemical inheritance. I have seen people make significant changes in the way they typically respond by learning how to turn round self-defeating attitudes and develop self-help techniques such as relaxation.

Your personality

There are some personality traits that are regarded as special risk factors for distress:

- A constant drive to succeed and excessive fear of failure.
- Ultra-competitiveness.
- A tendency to react excessively to any real or perceived loss of control by becoming highly emotional, and either striving to regain control or despairing and giving up in great frustration.
- Hostility and aggressiveness toward others (which may be hidden and expressed in competitiveness).
- Preferring work to recreation and socialising; feeling guilty when on holiday or not working.
- Tension, restlessness, impatience and irritability, especially when things seem to be happening slowly.
- A sense of being highly pressured by time and what has to be done; always rushing around, doing everything rapidly, finding it hard to be still.

These tendencies often lead to problems such as sleep disturbance, indigestion, increased risk of heart disease[5] and difficulties with relationships both at and away from work.

Type A or type B?

Many of the characteristics described above are typical of what has been called the Type A personality. This is in contrast to the Type B personality, which is more easygoing, less competitive and less concerned with failure or loss of control. Type Bs can be just as ambitious, work just as hard and be in equally stressful environments, but are less likely to give up when frustrated and suffer fewer of the harmful effects of stress.

These types are, of course, generalisations. In reality, most people fit somewhere between the two. Type A traits tend to be most pronounced in leaders, executives and senior managers. They are also more likely to be found in men, though this may change as more women enter management positions and ideas about women's roles and place in society continue to change. This is not to say that either the Type A or Type B personality is simply a result of cultural learning; they are more probably a combination of biology *and* culture.

External locus of control

Many people see themselves as being controlled by outside forces such as luck, chance or fate; or powers beyond their personal control like 'the system'; or by fixed personal traits that are unchangeable. Such people experience higher levels of stress than those who believe they have control over their feelings and at least partial control over the events that shape their lives.[6]

The externally controlled person typically acts and reacts in a number of ways that increase their risk of distress:[7]

- They use 'they' language, talk of 'unfairness' or 'unjustness', see self as a 'victim'.
- They are inclined to fear death (both their own and that of people close to them).
- They become overly distressed when exposed to unwanted events or circumstances.
- They have low resistance to infectious diseases and a shorter life expectancy, are generally more susceptible to illness, and show the effects of ageing at an early stage.
- They recover slowly after medical episodes, tending to avoid their usual activities for long periods and trust recovery to luck.
- They have a tendency to depression.
- They are inclined to choose activities involving luck more than skill.
- They have a low achievement level.
- They fail to engage in problem-solving behaviour to change disliked circumstances.

Lack of self-acceptance

Do you have trouble accepting yourself? This can lead to a number of stress-related problems:

- *Lack of self-knowledge.* You may deny (to yourself as well as others) unhelpful characteristics you would be better facing up to and changing.
- *Ego anxiety.* You may feel emotional tension when you believe that your self or personal worth is threatened, or that you must perform well or be approved of by others. This can be a powerful, even overwhelming, sensation. It is often accompanied by feelings of inadequacy, guilt, shame and possibly depression.
- *Avoidance.* You may — through fear of self-downing — avoid taking responsibility for problems.
- *Lack of confidence.* If you don't trust your own judgement, you will find it hard to make decisions or take risks.
- *Overconcern with status, approval and disapproval.* You may look to other people to accept you, and become anxious at any hint of disapproval.
- *Unassertive behaviour.* Fear of what others may think will make it hard to ask for what you want and say no to what you don't.

What causes lack of self-acceptance? There is one main underlying cause: a belief that you *should* be something other than what you are.

This demand originates in a natural human tendency to wish to improve oneself. This in turn probably has its origin in the evolutionary advantage of increasing one's chances of survival.

Sitting on this base, though, will be many years of learning. You may have been told time and again that you should be better than you are. You may have observed and modelled yourself on a parent who was never satisfied with him- or herself. Perhaps you had experiences while growing up that you interpreted as proof of your badness or uselessness as a person. Consequently, your inherent (and functional) *desire* continually to improve yourself has become an absolute *demand*.

Low tolerance: the ultimate predisposition?

There is one final predisposition that, I suspect, is the most common underlying cause of distress. Paradoxically, it seems to be the one of which people are least conscious. According to a concept developed by psychologist Albert

Ellis, low tolerance arises from believing that frustration and discomfort are intolerable and must therefore be avoided at all costs.

What is low tolerance?

Low tolerance comes in two slightly different but related flavours:

1. *Low frustration tolerance (LFT)* is caused by 'catastrophising' about being frustrated and demanding that it not happen. It is based on beliefs like:
   – 'The world owes me contentment and happiness.'
   – 'Things should be as I want them to be, and I can't stand it when they aren't.'
   – 'It's intolerable to be frustrated, so I must avoid it at all costs.'
   – 'Other people shouldn't do things that frustrate me.'
2. *Low discomfort tolerance (LDT)* arises from catastrophising about discomfort (including the discomfort of negative emotions) and demanding that it be avoided. It is based on beliefs like:
   – 'I should be able to feel happy all of the time.'
   – 'I must be able to feel comfortable all of the time.'
   – 'Discomfort and pain are awful and intolerable, and I must avoid them at all costs.'
   – 'I must not feel bad.'
   – 'I must have certainty in my life.'

These two types of low tolerance are similar and closely related. Frustration is uncomfortable, and discomfort is frustrating. Often, one term is used to refer to both types.

How low tolerance creates distress

Low tolerance contributes to distress in two main ways: first by creating it directly, and second by blocking the distressed person from using stress-management strategies.

- *Discomfort anxiety* is the emotional tension that results when people believe their comfort (or life) is threatened, that they should or must get what they want (and not get what they don't want), and that it is awful and unbearable (rather than merely inconvenient or disadvantageous) when things don't happen as they 'must'.
- *Worrying* is based on the belief: 'Because . . . would be awful, and I couldn't stand it, I must worry about it in case it happens.'

- *Avoidance.* If events and circumstances are seen as intolerable, too hard to bear and too difficult to overcome, a person is likely to develop the demand that they be avoided. However, it is in our interests to undergo some difficult experiences, such as grief after a loss, or the discomfort of personal change. Avoidance will only create greater problems later on.
- *Secondary disturbance.* This is the common human tendency to have a problem about having a problem. People often make themselves anxious about being anxious, depressed about being depressed, anxious about feeling guilty, and guilty about feeling angry. Secondary problems about stress result from:
  - Awfulising: 'Stress is dreadful.'
  - Discomfort intolerance: 'I can't bear to be stressed.'
  - Demanding: 'I must not/should not have to experience stress', or 'I should be able to handle stress better.'
  - Self-downing: 'Because I can't handle stress, I'm (useless, hopeless, no good, weak, etc.).'

  If you worry about being stressed, demand you not get stressed, or put yourself down for feeling stressed, you will make yourself *more* stressed!
- *Short-range enjoyment.* Another common human tendency, short-range enjoyment is the seeking of immediate pleasure or avoidance of pain at the cost of long-term stress. Examples include the abuse of alcohol, drugs and food, watching television at the expense of exercising, practising unsafe sex, or overspending to feel better.
- *Procrastination.* Short-range enjoyment and the avoidance of discomfort may cause you to put off difficult tasks or dealing with unpleasant situations — which leads to more stress in the long run.
- *Addictive tendencies.* Low tolerance is a key factor in the development of addictions.[8] To resist the impulse of the moment and go without is 'too uncomfortable' or 'frustrating'. It seems easier to give in to the urge to misuse alcohol, take drugs, gamble, or exercise obsessively. Much addictive behaviour serves to help people avoid pain. Most substance abusers are, in effect, medicating themselves to get rid of bad feelings. Unfortunately, once this tendency is established, it is hard to give up. Addictions create stress in the long run through damage to the body, strained relationships and the distress of withdrawal.

- *Negativity and complaining.* Low tolerance may cause you to become distressed over small hindrances and setbacks, overconcerned with unfairness, and prone to make comparisons between your own and others' circumstances. Negativity tends to alienate others, resulting in the loss of their support.
- *Failure to use stress management skills.* Low tolerance is a key reason people may learn strategies for managing stress but give up using them.

Overcoming your predispositions

List what you think may be your top three predispositions to stress. These are the things to be aware of and give special attention to as you learn how to deal with stress:

1. _____
   _____
2. _____
   _____
3. _____
   _____

There are certain aspects of ourselves that, with our present state of knowledge, we cannot change. But even when they are part of our genetic inheritance or personality, we can learn how to live around them. Remember that the main determinant of how you feel and behave is your belief system and what you think about yourself, others and the world. You can choose to change those beliefs. Neither your inherited nor your learned characteristics need totally control your life.

Further reading on the causes of stress

Carducci, Bernardo J., and Zimbardo, Philip G. 'Are You Shy?'. *Psychology Today*, 28:6 (Nov–Dec), 34–82, 1995.
Carpi, John. 'Stress: It's Worse Than You Think'. *Psychology Today*, 29:1 (Jan–Feb), 34–70, 1996.
Seligman, Martin E.P. *What You Can Change and What You Can't: The complete guide to successful self-improvement.* Random House, Sydney, 1994.

5
The Importance of Your Belief System

Your biological inheritance and past learning set the scene, but what determines your reactions to stress triggers in the present are the beliefs you carry with you now. Later we will examine how to identify and change self-defeating beliefs, but the first step is knowing what to look for. Accordingly, Part One concludes by outlining the nature of self-defeating thinking.

Thinking and stress

Whether or not a stress trigger affects you will depend on your assessment of it. You will experience stress if you believe that something is placing demands on your resources and is a threat to your physical or emotional comfort, self-image or lifestyle.

Your assessment may be accurate or distorted. Your body may become aroused when it doesn't need to — because you perceive danger when it doesn't exist or you overestimate it. It is also possible to be underaroused and fail to recognise a real danger — for example, the danger of driving after drinking alcohol.

How do you view life and stress?

There are a number of factors which affect how you view life and stress:

- Your beliefs about where personal control is located — externally or internally.
- How you view yourself.
- Your beliefs about the world.
- Your values and goals.
- Your level of commitment (the greater your commitment to something, the greater the potential for threat or challenge).

Your beliefs, values and level of commitment together determine how you interpret and evaluate events and your competence to deal with them.

Beliefs and biological predispositions

Your belief system sits on top of your biological inheritance. To some extent, what you believe is influenced by the type of temperament you have. If, for example, you see the world as a dangerous place, an inclination towards high arousability will exacerbate this.

On the other hand, beliefs can weaken the influence of your temperament. If a high-arousal person learns to reinterpret their feelings as merely uncomfortable rather than catastrophic, they can learn to be less reactive to them.

What is self-defeating thinking?

Most of your beliefs will probably be quite functional for you, or at least not harmful (even when they are less than totally accurate or logical!). You need be concerned only with those beliefs and attitudes that are self-defeating — the ones that lead to unnecessary personal disturbance and block you from achieving your goals. Such beliefs usually have the following characteristics:

1. They distort reality.
2. They are illogical:
   - they exaggerate the badness of events and circumstances
   - they are expressed in terms of absolute 'shoulds' and 'musts'
   - they make absolute judgements of people (including yourself)
3. They result in severe or extreme emotions that may be disabling and block you from achieving your goals.

The three levels of thinking

Thinking, whether it is self-defeating or rational, occurs on three levels: (1) *interpretations* of reality, (2) *evaluations* of those interpretations, and (3) *underlying rules* that ultimately determine the interpretations and evaluations.

Interpretations

Interpretations are the inferences we make about reality — that is, supposedly factual statements about what has happened, is happening or might happen.

Faulty interpretations are conclusions about a situation that have been drawn prematurely, without a full understanding of the situation. There are seven ways in which we might misinterpret events and circumstances.

Tick any that you recognise as typical of yourself:

Type	*Example*
☐ *Black and white thinking.* Viewing things in extremes, with no middle ground (also known as *all-or-nothing thinking*).	1. 'Because I forgot to say . . . , my whole lecture was a flop.'
☐ *Filtering.* Seeing all that is wrong while ignoring (filtering out) the positives.	2. 'There's nothing good about this restructuring.'
☐ *Overgeneralising.* Assuming that one event or circumstance represents the situation in total; or that something is happening 'all the time' or will happen 'forever'.	3. 'Everything's going wrong in my life.'
☐ *Mind-reading.* Jumping to conclusions, without evidence, about what other people are thinking.	4. 'She said that because she hates me.'
☐ *Fortune-telling.* Treating beliefs about the future as realities rather than predictions.	5. 'We'll end up in debt now that overtime has been cut.'
☐ *Emotional reasoning.* Believing that because you *feel* a certain way, that is how it really *is*.	6. 'I know she was out to get me, otherwise why would I feel so upset about it?'
☐ *Personalising.* Jumping to the conclusion, without evidence, that an event or circumstance is directly connected with you.	7. 'He was referring to me when he said the office was getting slack.'

Irrational interpretations usually result from holding self-defeating rules (as we shall see shortly).

Evaluations

As well as interpreting events and circumstances, we evaluate, or rate, them. (To be strictly correct, we evaluate our interpretations of them.) There are four types of evaluation that are stress-inducing. Tick those most characteristic of yourself:

- ☐ *Awfulising* — It's awful/terrible/horrible.
- ☐ *Discomfort intolerance* — It's unbearable. I can't stand it.
- ☐ *Demanding* — Things shouldn't be as they are. That must/mustn't happen.
- ☐ *People-rating* (including *self-rating*) — They're no good. I'm no good.

Here are some examples of stress-inducing evaluations (using the interpretations in the previous table):

Interpretation	*Possible evaluation*
1. Because I forgot to say . . . , my whole lecture was a flop.	I'm useless. (*People-rating*)
2. There's nothing good about this restructuring.	This shouldn't be happening. (*Demanding*)
3. Everything's going wrong in my life.	I can't stand it. (*Discomfort intolerance*)
4. She said that because she hates me.	I must be a total bastard for anyone to think so badly of me for what I did. (*Self-rating*)
5. We'll end up in debt now that overtime has been cut.	That will be terrible. (A*wfulising*)
6. I know she was out to get me, otherwise why would I feel so upset about it?	She shouldn't have done what she did. (*Demanding*)
7. He was referring to me when he said the office was getting slack.	It's horrible to be treated this way. (*Awfulising*)

Evaluations follow from the interpretations we make. Like interpretations, they pertain to specific situations but are determined by the general rules we follow.

Underlying rules

Our rules underlie our interpretations and their subsequent evaluations. They are a set of beliefs and attitudes that are general, global and reasonably enduring. They are with us all the time, albeit in our subconscious. Here are some examples of stress-inducing rules that may underlie the evaluations listed above:

1. 'My performance determines what kind of person I am.'
2. 'Life must always be safe and predictable.'
3. 'Discomfort and pain are unbearable.'
4. 'When I behave badly, this says something about me as a person.'
5. 'I must get disturbed about things that go wrong, otherwise the worst could happen.'
6. 'I must always be treated fairly.'
7. 'It's awful to be criticised.'

Note how rules are stated in general terms. Each will apply to many situations. The *general* rules we hold determine how we interpret and evaluate *specific* situations. Our underlying rules determine our personality, our tolerance for frustration and discomfort, our level of self-confidence, how assertive we are, and whether we are externally or internally directed.

Because of the defining role our rules play in how we view the world and react to it, time spent analysing them is time well spent. How you can do this is a key focus of Part Two.

Further reading on thinking and stress

Bernard, Michael E. *Staying Rational in an Irrational World: Albert Ellis and Rational-Emotive Therapy.* Lyle Stuart, New York, 1986.
Ellis, Albert. *How to Stubbornly Refuse to Make Yourself Miserable About Anything.* Lyle Stuart, New York, 1988.

Part Two

The Foundations for Effective Stress Management

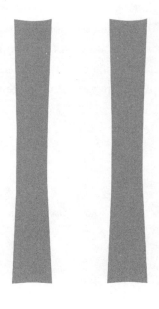

Part One examined the causes of stress, how to recognise its symptoms, and the nature of self-defeating thinking. Part Two considers how stress can be managed. First, it looks at what doesn't work, and what does. Then it introduces the *Twelve Rational Principles*. These principles form the heart of the book. Applying them makes it possible to overcome the common blocks to stress-management strategies. Part Two finishes with a description of *Rational Effectiveness Training* — a set of techniques you can use to move the twelve principles from your head to your feet.

6
How You Can Make Stress Management Work

To put into practice better ways of doing something, we first need to identify and get rid of the old ways. Unfortunately, many people use methods of managing stress which represent solutions that are worse than the problem. Such methods involve reactions that are out of proportion to the trigger, don't meet the demands of the situation, and are destructive to the user and other people.

What works and what doesn't

Dysfunctional coping methods are usually designed either to avoid the stress trigger, or to get rid of the bad feelings involved, or both. Here is a list of the more common ones to watch out for. Tick any you tend to use:

☐ *Aggression*
Screaming, shouting, threatening, verbally abusing, belittling or passively making things difficult, are intended to control the behaviour of other people. Aggressive acts of this kind, though, often have stressful results — people may retaliate or withdraw their support.

☐ *Apathy*
To do nothing may bring short-term security and avoid discomfort. Unfortunately, however, it reinforces low tolerance, maintains unpleasant situations and leads to suppressed resentment.

☐ *Unassertiveness*
Not speaking up, not asking for what you want, or standing back from difficult situations also serve the purpose of avoidance. But they reinforce low tolerance, cause people to lose respect for you, and change nothing.

☐ *Indecision*
Not deciding avoids the risk of making a wrong decision. But as well as reinforcing low tolerance, it causes opportunities to be lost and leaves problems unresolved.

☐ *Procrastination*

Putting off difficult tasks, issues and decisions is yet another way to put off discomfort. The problem is, things mount up, nothing changes, and low tolerance is again reinforced.

☐ *Overinvolvement*

Becoming obsessed with an activity — be it work, a sport or a hobby — may be a way of avoiding an unpleasant reality, such as a relationship problem. Unfortunately, the obsession can become a problem in its own right — and the original problem is still there.

☐ *Perfectionism*

Rigidly applying rules and instructions, putting off unpleasant tasks or spending excessive time on them may serve the purpose of avoiding difficulties or minimising the risk of failure. Unfortunately, as David Burns has shown in 'The Perfectionist's Script for Self-Defeat',[1] perfectionism also reduces efficiency and output.

☐ *Blaming*

Acknowledging your own failings and imperfections can be avoided by blaming others, but this only reinforces low tolerance and results in failure to learn from mistakes.

☐ *Nostalgia*

Longing for a return to 'the good old days' is another way to avoid current realities. But problems mount up, life goes on without you, and you have less and less control.

☐ *Worrying*

People worry mostly because they think it will stop a problem happening. But the worrying itself creates distress — whether or not the anticipated problem actually materialises — and with attention diverted from problem-solving, bad things are more likely to occur!

☐ *Addictive behaviour*

People often try to self-medicate their bad feelings by using alcohol, tranquillisers, sleeping pills or illegal drugs, by overeating or eating unhealthy food, or by overexercising. Unfortunately, such behaviour can become addictive and a problem in itself, causing greater pain in the long run. Meanwhile, the original problems continue to mount up.

What to do instead

Now that we have listed the unhelpful responses to avoid, let us replace them with what works. If you were to look through books or descriptions of training programmes on stress management, you would most likely see a list of topics like the one below. This itemises the standard stress-management strategies, which Part Three looks at in detail. Tick those on which you think you need to do some work:

- ☐ Have clear and realistic goals.
- ☐ Look after your body.
- ☐ Be able to relax your body and mind.
- ☐ Sleep well.
- ☐ Maintain a support system.
- ☐ Act assertively in your dealings with others.
- ☐ Keep stimulation and variety in your life.
- ☐ Manage time to achieve your goals.
- ☐ Manage your financial and material resources.
- ☐ Manage the changes in your life.
- ☐ Know how to problem-solve.
- ☐ Ask for help when you need it.

Which of the strategies you have ticked are priorities for you to work on? Record the top four here:

1._____
2._____
3._____
4._____

Why it often doesn't work

The strategies in the list above all probably appear as common sense to you. Unfortunately, it seems that people often know about them but fail to put them into practice, or give them up before they have had a chance to work. Why is this? From my work with distressed people over the years, I have identified a number of principal reasons.

The training may be faulty

Programmes and books are often presented as 'one size fits all'. They do not take into account that different people have different problems, differing values and a variety of coping styles.

You are unlikely to employ strategies that are at odds with your values. Let's say, for example, that you are encouraged to express your anger rather than hold it in. If you have been brought up to believe that anger is 'evil', you may not be inclined to follow this advice; or if you do, you may create a new problem — guilt — which is likely to make you give up.

Nor are you likely to use strategies that clash with your coping style. If, for example, you are a physically active person, being told to relax with a novel is unlikely to work.

This book will help you develop a better understanding of your own values and coping style, and show you how to develop stress-management strategies that are compatible with them.

There may be blocks within yourself

Unfortunately, many programmes ignore the most common block to the effective use of stress-management strategies — self-defeating thinking. As we saw in Part One, self-defeating beliefs (1) distort reality, (2) are illogical, and (3) result in extreme, possibly disabling, emotions which prevent you achieving your goals.

There are probably as many self-defeating beliefs as there are people in the world, but we can usefully summarise them under twelve main headings. Tick the ones you think are problematical for you:

☐ *Lack of self-knowledge*
You place a low priority on having clear values and goals and knowing your abilities and limits.

☐ *Low confidence and lack of self-acceptance*
You see approval and recognition (and avoidance of disapproval) as absolute necessities; believe your performance determines what kind of person you are, and that you must succeed at whatever you do and never make significant mistakes; and don't trust yourself or your judgements.

☐ *Unbalanced self-interest*
You think you don't matter, so consider other people's wants as more important than your own and always put them first; or, at the other extreme, you believe other people's feelings, goals and wants are of no relevance to you at all.

☐ *Low tolerance for frustration and discomfort*
You believe you must feel good all the time; that life should be easy and you shouldn't have to work hard at coping with it; that other people or things should change rather than you; that discomfort and pain are intolerable and must be avoided at all costs; that to feel happy, you must always be in control of yourself and your circumstances and have things the way you want.

☐ *Short-range enjoyment*

You think you should be able to satisfy your wants immediately and regard it as intolerable to have to wait.

☐ *Overcautiousness*

You believe you can be better off by avoiding life's difficulties, unpleasantness and responsibilities; that you must avoid any risk of things going wrong in your life; that you can only avoid bad events by worrying about them; and that you must always ensure you succeed at whatever you do and never make significant mistakes.

☐ *Excessiveness*

You consider having less than what you want to be unbearably frustrating, and that to feel OK you must go to the limit in whatever you do.

☐ *Emotional and behavioural irresponsibility*

You believe that how you feel and behave are controlled by forces outside you, or are the result of events in your past, so there is nothing much you can do to feel better or alter your behaviour.

☐ *External-directedness and lack of commitment*

You think you need people who are stronger than you to prop you up and show you what to do with your life; that you can be happier by just drifting through life with only superficial commitments; or that you could not stand losing anything important to you, so you must avoid becoming too committed to anything.

☐ *Inflexibility*

You believe there is always a 'right' and 'wrong' way to do things; and that people should always do the right thing and must be blamed and corrected when they behave wrongly.

☐ *Magical thinking*

You think that believing in something makes it true; that what is true now will be true forever; that there are ultimate truths which can never be challenged and which will never change; and that there are external forces such as 'fate' that control your life and destiny.

☐ *Demanding that reality not exist*

You believe the world should always be a just and fair place, and that highly undesirable events should not occur.

These self-defeating ways of thinking are major blocks to effective stress management. The next chapter explores twelve rational alternatives.

What stress management is really about

We don't eliminate stress — we manage it

Get rid of any idea that if you learn stress management you will be cured for life and never have to combat stress again. Such a notion will only lead to disillusionment. What you can do, however, is acquire some skills which you can then apply as and when you *choose* to.

Stress management involves using strategies that will help you control stress symptoms, function better in everyday life and influence what happens to you. Although these strategies will become more habitual as time goes by, you will still need to use them, often consciously and deliberately, throughout your life.

Good management attends to triggers, consequences and attitudes

It is possible to address an external stress trigger but at great internal cost — for example, by saying no to an unreasonable demand but feeling guilty as a consequence. This is not good management.

On the other hand, attending to the symptoms of distress but not the trigger may not be good management either — like using alcohol to alleviate bad feelings about a destructive relationship.

What is good management? Good management involves taking action aimed at both the external trigger and your internal reactions or symptoms. Most importantly, however, it involves dealing with the beliefs that come between the two and ultimately determine how you feel and behave.

What is rational thinking?

Rational beliefs have the following characteristics:

1. They are consistent with the real world.
2. They are logical:
   – they keep the badness of events and circumstances in perspective
   – they stress preferential thinking rather than absolute demands
   – they judge behaviour rather than people
3. They result in moderate rather than extreme emotions and facilitate the achievement of personal goals.

Making stress management work for you

To summarise, there are four prerequisites for effective stress management:

1. You have detected any 'clinical' conditions (such as depression, anxiety or any of the others described in Chapter 2) that may prevent you from effectively managing stress.
2. You are clear about which of the standard stress-management skills (described in detail in Part Three) you could usefully develop.
3. You know how to identify and change self-defeating thinking when you feel distressed (Chapter 8 will show you how to do this).
4. You know how to systematically replace self-defeating attitudes with more functional principles to guide your reactions to specific events and circumstances and your life in general. The next chapter looks at twelve such principles.

7
The Twelve Rational Principles

The twelve principles outlined below form the heart of this book. They provide a basis for achieving success in stress management in two ways. First, they will enable you to counter the self-defeating beliefs that create distress. Second, they will help you overcome common blocks to using the practical strategies that are a standard part of stress-management training.

Self-knowledge

Self-knowledge appears as the first principle, because most of the others build on it. It involves knowing your capabilities and your limits, your personal temperament and typical coping style, and your values and goals.

Aspects of self-knowledge

Are you what Hans Selye calls a 'racehorse', or are you a 'turtle'?[1] Racehorses thrive on stress and are only happy with a vigorous, fast-paced lifestyle. Turtles require peace, quiet and a generally tranquil environment. These are, of course, extremes — people usually fall somewhere in between.

What are your values? What matters to you? Where do you stand on issues of the day? What do you want to achieve in life? Though you will share many aspects with others in your social group, every person has a unique system of values and goals.

Everyone has certain abilities — and limits. Do you recognise your abilities and make the most of them? Do you also acknowledge your limits and know when to stop?

Why knowing yourself is important to stress management

You may feel comfortable with some of your characteristics, less happy with others. In either case, to manage stress effectively you need to be aware of your own optimum stress level and coping style, as well as the goals and values that guide your reactions.

Everyone has their own temperament, style of managing stress and value system. The strategies you develop need to be relevant to your personal style and compatible with your personal values, otherwise you are not likely to use them.

Developing self-knowledge

How can you become more aware of your coping style and optimum stress level? Here are some suggestions:

- Identify those stress triggers that typically affect you. In what situations do you tend to feel stressed? You could use the list on pages 27–30 as a prompt. Better still, keep a log for a few weeks.
- You are the best intuitive judge of your optimum stress level. Observe what your body is doing; note your characteristic stress signs. See the list on pages 22–4. Which of these symptoms do you recognise in yourself? Include these in your log.
- Observe how you usually cope with problems. What works for you? What do you tend to do that is unhelpful? Do you identify with any of the dysfunctional coping methods listed on pages 47–8?
- Strategies for identifying personal values and goals are listed on pages 96–100. Use these to check out your preferences, values and standards. Are they realistic and appropriate? Have you thought them through for yourself?
- Employing *Rational Self-Analysis* (p. 80) will help you identify the underlying values that prompt your reactions to specific events and circumstances.

Self-acceptance and confidence

Self-acceptance and confidence are closely related concepts. One builds on the other. Being able to accept yourself as you are, free of any demand that you be different, provides the basis for confidence in your abilities. Confidence, in turn, enables you to take risks, try new things and direct your own life.

Accepting yourself

To accept yourself is to acknowledge three things: (1) you exist, (2) there is no reason why you should be any different from how you are, and (3) you are neither worthy nor unworthy.

1. To acknowledge that you exist is probably straightforward. It is the other two aspects that most people find hard to grasp.
2. Self-acceptance involves rejection of any *demand* that you be different. You may sensibly *prefer* to be different. You may decide it is *in your interests* to change some things. But keep the desire to change as a *preference*. Instead of believing that you *have* to change, see change as a *choice*.
3. Do not attempt to measure your self or set some kind of value on it. Self-acceptance is radically different from self-esteem. *Self-esteem* is based on the idea that you are a 'good' or 'worthwhile' person. Worthwhileness requires criteria, such as how well you perform, or an underpinning concept, e.g. that you are worthwhile simply because you exist. *Self-acceptance*, on the other hand, is based on the idea that you don't have to be 'good' or 'worthwhile'. In fact, there is no need to evaluate your *self* at all! Instead, use your energy and time to evaluate (1) your *behaviour,* and (2) the quality of your *existence*. By evaluating your behaviour, you can check whether it helps you enjoy your life and achieve your goals. By evaluating the quality of your existence, you can assess your level of enjoyment and achievement — more important, surely, than worrying about whether you are a 'worthwhile' person.

Having confidence in your abilities

Self-knowledge and self-acceptance are preconditions for confidence. There are three aspects to having confidence in your abilities: (1) you know what you can and cannot do; (2) you are prepared to try things to the limit of your ability; and (3) you work regularly at extending your capabilities.

Having confidence in your *abilities* is different from having confidence in your *self*. *Self*-confidence implies perfection — that you, as a *total* person, are able to do everything well. This is unrealistic and grandiose.

Having confidence in your *abilities* is more realistic. Instead of talking about self-confidence, follow the advice of Paul Hauck[2] and think in terms of social confidence, work confidence, driving confidence, house-care confidence, examination confidence, relationship confidence, and so on. In other words, develop confidence in specific abilities rather than in your total self.

In practice, *ability*-confidence involves behaviours like the following:

- Doing things without demanding you succeed, and viewing mistakes as opportunities for learning. Confidence grows out of the *attempt*, the doing, rather than from the *result*.

- Evaluating your actions and performances in terms of how they help you reach your goals — not what they 'prove' about you as a person.
- Taking calculated risks with important activities such as choosing a career, changing jobs or starting a new relationship.
- Persevering — not giving up when you do less well than you want; rejecting the belief that 'everything should come easy'; and accepting that many goals are reached only after overcoming obstacles and setbacks, and persisting over a period of time.
- Learning from experience — trying something, analysing what happened, seeing where you went wrong and working out what you can do to improve your abilities.

Why self-acceptance and confidence are important to stress management

If you are prone to rating your total self, you may want to avoid looking closely at your actions because to do so may lead to self-downing. Paradoxically, self-acceptance is more likely than self-evaluation to lead to constructive change. Confidence in your abilities will free you to take risks, try new experiences and learn new lessons.

If you can accept yourself, with your unique characteristics and preferences, you will be less likely to live your life to suit other people.

As Martin Seligman has pointed out, there are limits to how much we can change ourselves.[3] Human beings are not perfectible. If you can accept imperfection in yourself, you are less likely to engage in dangerous behaviour by striving for the unattainable.

Developing self-acceptance and confidence

Self-acceptance as an alternative to self-evaluation is not an easy concept to grasp. The human tendency to self-evaluate seems to be in-built, and the self-esteem concept is pervasive in our thinking and culture.

- Think through the philosophy of self-acceptance. Read about it. Write down your thoughts on it. Talk about it with others (many people will argue against the concept, which will give you the opportunity to hone your thinking!).
- Most importantly, *behave* like a self-accepting and confident person. As far as possible, *practise* living in accordance with your preferences,

values and standards. Say what you believe; be open and honest as to who you are (although do so appropriately, taking into account the preferences and feelings of others). Treat yourself to things you have tended to think you don't 'deserve'. Try things you have been afraid to do — without placing any demand on yourself that you succeed.

Enlightened self-interest

The ability to act in your own interests follows from self-acceptance and confidence. As we shall see, it is also important to take into account the interests of others. The principle of enlightened self-interest takes into account both aspects:

1. You place your own interests first.
2. You keep in mind that your own interests will be best served if you take into account the interests of others.

Human beings are fundamentally self-interested

Notwithstanding any precepts that say we 'should' be otherwise, human beings appear to be intrinsically concerned first and foremost with their own welfare.

Hans Selye has argued that the desire to maintain oneself and stay happy is the most ancient impulse that motivates living beings — and one of the most important for survival.[4] All living beings protect their own interests first of all. Selye points out that this begins with our basic biological make-up, in that the various cells in our bodies also act to ensure their own survival.

Human beings are also motivated by social interest

Selye has pointed out, though, that we are also strongly motivated by altruistic feelings. As well as *self*-interest, we are also driven by *social* interest — the wish to ensure that the social system as a whole survives and develops.

How is it that two apparently contradictory tendencies can coexist? The answer is that we help others in order to help ourselves. In other words, our self-interest is *enlightened*.

It appears that, like self-interest, social interest is also inherent within human beings and has biological roots. Body cells cooperate with each other. Collaboration enables the total organism to function, which in turn guarantees the survival of each individual cell.

In effect, *individual* interests are best served by *mutual* cooperation. Accordingly, self-interest without social interest is misguided. So is social interest without self-interest. Always putting others first can lead to resentment or a 'martyr' attitude. People who believe they are acting purely in the interests of others are dangerous. By denying (to themselves) that their own self-interest is involved, such people may justify all types of manipulative and controlling behaviour toward others.

People are both self-interested and socially interested. This dual tendency is built into our very being and begins with our basic biology. By accepting this about yourself, you will be able to do a better job of acting in your own interests — in an enlightened manner.

What is it to be 'enlightened'?

The word *enlightened* has several layers of meaning. One sense is *humanitarian* — charitable, liberal, idealistic. Another is *utilitarian* — useful, beneficial, practical.

Can you see how merging an enlightened attitude with innate self-interest can apply at all levels — to yourself, to your family, to your local community, to your country, and to the world as a whole? Consider the effect if every person on the planet acknowledged their self-interest and then practised it in an enlightened manner. What if every country based its external and foreign policies on the humanitarian and practical principle of enlightened self-interest?

Why enlightened self-interest is important to stress management

If human beings did not have an inherent will to protect themselves and further their own interests, they would not survive. If you don't attend to your own interests, who will? Knowing what is in your interests will help you get what is best for you and avoid what is harmful. It will keep you moving toward your goals — and ensure that your goals are the right ones for you.

But, simultaneously, you had better take into account the interests of others. Getting people to have positive feelings toward you is a good idea. They will be more likely to treat you well and less likely to harm you. Contributing to their welfare will encourage them to contribute to yours. And contributing to the development and survival of the society in which you live will mean a better environment in which to pursue your interests.

If you acknowledge that self-interest is inherent in your nature, you will feel less guilty about looking after yourself. If you acknowledge that altruistic behaviour is in your interests, you will be more likely to cooperate with others. If you do both, everyone gains.

Developing enlightened self-interest

Begin by practising enlightened behaviours. When you have trouble deciding what is in your interests, use the *benefits calculation* technique described on page 86. Here are some ideas to get you started now:

- Go out of your way to show positive feelings toward others — gratitude, respect, trust — which in turn will arouse goodwill from them.
- Choose some new activities in various areas of your life — at work, with your family, in your leisure pursuits — that will generate goodwill in others.
- At the same time, act assertively. Ask for what you want, say no to what you don't, and tell others (when appropriate) what you think and how you feel.
- For a while, make a point of doing something each day just for yourself.

Until enlightened self-interest becomes second nature, *consciously* seek to get more of what you want while facilitating the interests of the other people in your life.

Tolerance for frustration and discomfort

The ability to tolerate frustration and discomfort is central to stress management. High tolerance will keep you from overreacting to things you dislike. It will help you tackle problems and issues rather than avoid them. It will enable you to take risks and try new experiences.

What is high tolerance?

As we saw in Chapter 4, low tolerance for frustration and discomfort is a key cause of unnecessary distress. It arises from beliefs such as: 'Life shouldn't be hard', 'It's awful and I can't stand it when it's hard', 'I must avoid pain, difficulties and frustrations.'

High tolerance, on the other hand, involves accepting the reality of frustration and discomfort and keeping their badness in perspective.

To accept frustration and discomfort is to acknowledge that, while you may dislike them, they are realities. They exist, and there is no Law of the Universe that says they 'shouldn't' exist (although you may *prefer* they didn't). You expect to experience *appropriate* negative emotions such as concern, remorse, regret, sadness, annoyance and disappointment; but you avoid exaggerating these emotions (by telling yourself you can't stand them) into anxiety, guilt, shame, depression, hostile anger and self-pity.

To keep frustration and discomfort in perspective is to regard them as unpleasant rather than awful. It is to dislike rejection, pain, bad health, financial insecurity and other unwanted circumstances, but to believe you can cope with the discomfort they cause when they arise.

Why high tolerance is important to stress management

Low tolerance creates distress by making a person overreact to discomfort. It may lead to *secondary problems* (having a problem about having a problem), a reaction to symptoms of distress which brings about additional symptoms. You might, for example, get angry because you feel uncomfortable, or become depressed because you feel anxious. Low tolerance also impedes the use of stress-management strategies such as changing one's diet, exercising, time management or acting assertively.

High tolerance, on the other hand, helps in many ways. Adopt it and you will be:

- Less likely to create secondary problems by overreacting to unwanted events and circumstances.
- More willing to experience present discomfort to achieve long-term goals and enjoyment.
- Prepared to take reasonable risks.
- More able to assert yourself appropriately with other people.
- Less likely to put off difficult tasks and issues, including personal change.

How to raise your tolerance for discomfort and frustration

- Know when you are engaging in low-tolerance behaviour aimed at avoiding discomfort or frustration. Keep a log of such behaviour for a period of several weeks or longer. Watch out for tendencies or habits like:
  – avoiding uncomfortable situations
  – overusing drugs or alcohol
  – compulsive gambling, shopping, exercising or bingeing on food
  – losing your temper
  – putting off difficult tasks
- The technique of *exposure* (p. 88) is the best way to increase your

tolerance. Make a list of things you typically avoid — situations, events, thoughts, risks, etc. Commit yourself to face at least one of these each day. Actively confront discomfort by entering uncomfortable situations. Instead of trying to escape the frustration or discomfort as you normally would, *stay with it* until it diminishes of its own accord.

- You can prepare yourself to cope with discomfort by using *Rational Self-Analysis* (p. 80), *imagery* (p. 86) and the *blow-up technique* (p. 87). Afterwards, do a *catastrophe scale* (p. 85) to get your reaction to the discomfort into perspective.

Long-range enjoyment

Like most people, you probably want to enjoy life. As well as avoiding distress, you want to experience pleasure. And you probably want pleasure now, not tomorrow. As Alice said in *Through the Looking-glass*: 'It must come sometimes to "jam today".'[5] But there are times when it is in our interests to forgo immediate pleasure in order to obtain greater enjoyment in the longer term.

What is long-range enjoyment?

There are two components to the principle of long-range enjoyment. One is the seeking of enjoyment in each and every present moment, rather than putting off pleasure until 'tomorrow', or dwelling on the past.

However, to ensure a continuation of enjoyable present moments, it is sometimes necessary to postpone pleasure. For example, you may wish to drink more alcohol now, but by restricting your intake today you will keep your body in shape for further consumption in ten years' time. Or you may wish to buy a new stereo, but instead make do with the one you already have and save the money for the greater pleasure of an overseas trip. This is the 'long-term' part.

The principle can be summed up as follows: *live for the present with an eye to the future.* In other words, seek as much pleasure and enjoyment as you can in the present while taking into account the desirability of enjoying your life in the long term.

The concept is not new

The underlying thinking behind the concept of long-range enjoyment has been around for thousands of years. The Greek philosopher Epicurus (341–

270 B.C.) proposed the idea that pleasure is the supreme good and main goal of life — *and* that only through self-restraint and moderation can people achieve true happiness.

John Stuart Mill, British philosopher and economist, argued that an act is right if it brings pleasure, and wrong if it brings pain. But he introduced the caveat that the ultimate value is the good of society, and the guiding principle of individual conduct is the welfare of the greatest number of people, so personal pleasure may sometimes be postponed for the sake of greater ends in the long run.

Developing long-range enjoyment

- Learn to calculate gains and losses. Weigh the short-term pleasurable effects of an action against its possible longer-term negative effects. Make sure that immediate gain doesn't set you up for future pain — as, for instance, with overindulgence in alcohol. If in doubt, do a *benefits calculation* (p. 86).
- Weigh short-term discomfort and frustration against the prospect of greater and more enduring comfort in the long term. To start exercising might well be more uncomfortable than watching television, but in the future not only will you feel the health benefits, you will actually begin to enjoy the exercise itself.
- The strategy of *paradoxical behaviour* (p. 89) will help you put your change of philosophy into action. Practise deliberately postponing gratification in order to increase your tolerance for frustration. List a few things you could go without and earmark the money you save for something you would really like. Take half an hour off your usual television-watching and exercise instead, and reward yourself with an occasional special treat. Be creative. What other ideas for practising long-range enjoyment can you come up with?

By now you will probably have begun to see that many of the twelve principles are interdependent. To delay gratification involves tolerating frustration. Long-range enjoyment of relationships will sometimes involve enlightened self-interest in your dealings with others, while moderation in your eating and drinking habits will benefit your health and quality of life in the long term.

To sum up

If you *always* postponed pleasure, you would never enjoy life. But if you *always* live for the present, your happiness and stress management in the future will eventually be compromised. Live your life in such a way that you get maximum enjoyment both now *and* in the future.

Risk-taking

Human beings, by nature, seek safety, predictability and freedom from fear. But humans also pursue risk. A totally secure life would be a boring one. To grow as a person and improve one's quality of life means being prepared to take some chances.

The principle

What this involves is a willingness to take sensible risks in order to get more out of life and avoid the distress of boredom, listlessness and dissatisfaction. Here are some important areas of risk-taking that relate to stress management:

- Considering new ideas which may challenge existing beliefs.
- Tackling tasks which offer no guarantee of success.
- Trying new relationships.
- Doing things that risk the disapproval of other people.

· Why risk-taking is relevant to stress management

Risk-taking is a prerequisite of self-knowledge. To discover your limits, you need to take some risks and try yourself out. In so doing you will open up fresh opportunities to increase pleasure and avoid boredom.

Problem-solving entails taking a chance on solutions that may backfire. To act assertively is to risk disapproval or rejection. Maintaining a support system involves trusting and opening up to other people.

Finally, experimenting with different activities to discover what you like and dislike will increase your self-knowledge and help you clarify your goals and values.

Increasing your willingness to take risks

- *Exposure* (p. 88) is a key risk-taking technique. Draw up a list of things you would like to try, such as:

– asking someone for something — like a date or favour — when there is a chance of rejection.

– doing something when there is a chance others will disapprove — for example, speaking up and telling a group of people what you think about an issue.

– trying something when there is no guarantee of success.

Put one item a day into practice. As you do so, remind yourself that the discomfort involved is not intolerable, and that staying with it will gradually increase your tolerance.

- A *benefits calculation* (p. 86) can help you make rational decisions about the usefulness of risks you are considering.
- You can prepare yourself for taking risks and cope with the discomfort involved using *Rational Self-Analysis* (p. 80), *coping rehearsal* (p. 87), the *blow-up technique* (p. 87) and *role-playing* (p. 90).

Moderation

Sensible risk-taking recognises the innate human desire for safety and security. The principle of moderation will help you avoid extremes in thinking, feeling and behaving.

Why moderation is important to stress management

Extreme expectations — those which are too high or too low — will set you up for either constant failure or a life of boredom.

Addictive or obsessional behaviour can take control of you, creating new distress. Unrestrained eating, drinking or exercising will stress your body and lead to long-term health complications.

Obsessive habits in areas as diverse as your work or your sexual behaviour can damage relationships as well as strain your body.

The principle of moderation

Taking a moderate approach to life ranges from one's ultimate goals to one's daily activities.

It is necessary to develop long-term goals, short-term objectives and tasks that will challenge you and move you forwards. But it is equally important that whatever you plan is achievable so you do not set yourself up for failure and disillusionment.

If, for example, you aim to maintain a certain weight, ensure you set a level appropriate to your age and other personal factors. Avoid any tasks or activities that are extreme — like going on a diet that promises massive weight loss in a short time. Not only will such an approach damage your health, but eventually you are likely to regain any weight you lose (probably even more), leaving you with a feeling of hopelessness. The best way to maintain an appropriate weight without stressing your body is not to go on a radical diet but to moderate your eating and drinking over the long term.

This sort of approach applies in most areas of life. By all means throw yourself into your work, play, exercise and sexual life, but avoid the stress of overinvolvement. Moderate, too, your self-help programme — commit yourself to personal change, but without obsessiveness.

Note that moderation does not preclude risk-taking (moderating your pursuit of security will help you avoid that!). But you can take risks without being foolhardy.

Developing a moderate approach to life

- Identify any areas of your life where you tend to behave excessively — eating, exercising, sexual activity, using your computer, etc. Note when you are demanding full satisfaction of your urges, or catastrophising about the frustration involved in restraint. Keeping a log will help you do this.
- Use the strategies of *exposure* (p. 88) and *paradoxical behaviour* (p. 89) to get into action. Set up a list of tasks, sorted according to difficulty, which will give you practice in behaving moderately. Set limits in each case to define what is moderate and what excessive, and commit yourself to keeping within those limits.
- Handle your frustration using *Rational Self-Analysis* (p. 80). The *benefits calculation* (p. 86) will help you see which areas of your life you would do best to moderate. Finally, if you are unable to change behaviour which has become addictive, seek professional help.

Emotional and behavioural responsibility

As we saw in Part One, people who view their emotions and behaviour as under their control are less prone to distress than people who see themselves as controlled by external forces. The principle of responsibility can help you take charge of your emotions, your actions, and in turn your life. This entails taking responsibility for (1) what you feel, and (2) how you act.

To be *emotionally responsible* is to believe that you create your own feelings in reaction to what life throws at you. You avoid blaming other people — your parents, partner, boss or anyone else — for how you feel.

Behavioural responsibility means accepting you cause your own actions and behaviour, and are not compelled to behave in any particular way.

The inner-controlled person

An inner-controlled person can be identified by characteristics like the following:

- *Uses 'I' language* — 'I think that…' or 'I would like you to…' rather than '*Everyone* knows that…' or '*You* should…'.
- *Tends to be assertive* when relating to other people, rather than passive or aggressive.
- *Gets on with life now* rather than dwelling on the past or dreaming about the future but doing nothing to make it happen.
- *Takes setbacks in their stride* rather than catastrophising or bemoaning fate.
- *Has a problem-solving approach* — when things go wrong, looks for possible solutions.
- *Does not rely on 'luck'* — believes that action and the application of skill are what make things happen, rather than luck or fate.

Limits to emotional and behavioural responsibility

While your emotions are mainly caused by what you believe, there are some exceptions. Biochemical changes, for example, can lead to emotional changes. (How you react to biochemical variations, though, will still depend on how you *view* what is happening in your body.)

While you can, largely, control your thoughts, it is unlikely that anyone could do so *perfectly*. Expecting flawlessness will only lead to discouragement and self-downing.

While you are largely responsible for the consequences of your actions, some outcomes will be outside your control. If, for example, you say no to a request, the person making it may be disappointed — an appropriate reaction. You would be responsible for this in that your refusal was the trigger. But what if that person became clinically depressed — an inappropriate overreaction? That would be their responsibility, not yours. You have no control over whether people choose to view your actions in ways that are rational or self-defeating.

Finally, an important point. Don't fall into the trap of *blaming* yourself because you are responsible for what you feel and do. Blame and responsibility are not the same thing. Blame is *moralistic*. It seeks not only to identify who is the cause of a problem, but also to condemn them. Responsibility, on the other hand, is *practical*. It seeks either to identify a cause so it can be dealt with, or to identify who needs to take action for the problem to be solved — irrespective of who or what caused it. Responsibility is concerned not with moralising, but with finding solutions.

Why responsibility is important to stress management

Suzanne Kobasa has conducted research on, as she calls them, 'hardy' people — those who appear to thrive on stress.[6] A key characteristic of such people is their belief that they are in control of their lives. They generally have better physical and mental health — are less affected by the ageing process, recover faster from medical episodes such as a heart attack or surgery, and are less likely to suffer from depression or anxiety.

If you take responsibility for your feelings and behaviours, you will avoid making yourself a victim or overreacting to what other people say or do. You will be able to change your own feelings even though the world does not change to suit you. Finally, you will have confidence in your ability to handle your feelings, whatever happens, which will free you to take risks and try new experiences.

Developing responsibility

- Use *Rational Self-Analysis* (p. 80) to identify and dispute any irresponsible thinking.
- Make a list of things you do that demonstrate irresponsibility — unassertive behaviour, dwelling on the past, catastrophising, letting problems drift in the hope something will 'come along'. Use the technique of *paradoxical behaviour* (p. 89) to act differently in these areas, taking responsibility for how you feel and behave.

Self-direction and commitment

Emotional and behavioural responsibility lay the basis for taking control of your life and committing yourself to action and involvement.

Self-direction

Taking responsibility for the direction of your life involves:

- Choosing your goals — making sure they are your own.
- Actively pursuing your goals rather than waiting and dreaming.
- Making your own decisions, even though you may seek opinions from others.
- Choosing to work at managing stress, developing your potential and changing things you dislike, rather than just drifting along or expecting a miracle to occur.
- Not condemning any *person* (including yourself) when things go wrong in your life, even though you or someone else may be responsible. Instead, you identify any *causes* and look for *solutions*.

Self-direction does not mean open opposition to or non-cooperation with others. You can keep self-direction on track by balancing it with other principles such as enlightened self-interest, long-range enjoyment, moderation and flexibility (p. 71).

There are several prerequisites for self-direction. First, you need to view what happens to you as *influenced* (but not totally controlled) by what you do. As we have seen, inner-controlled people tend to be assertive, get on with life and do not see themselves as victims. Second, to direct your own life you need to know what you want to do with it. Have you clarified your goals and values? Chapter 9 will show you how to do this.

Commitment

Commitment follows from self-direction. There are two elements:

1. *Perseverance.* This is the ability to bind yourself emotionally and intellectually to a course of action. It involves a willingness to do the necessary work (and tolerate the discomfort involved) to effect personal change and achieve goals.
2. *Deep involvement.* This is the ability to enjoy and become absorbed in (but not addicted to) other people, activities and interests as ends in themselves — to get pleasure from the *doing*, irrespective of the final result. It applies in all areas — work, home, sports, hobbies, creative activities and the world of ideas.

Limits to self-direction and commitment

Some of what happens to you will be out of your control, and this will place limits on how much you can influence events and outcomes. Remember, though, that how you *react* to those is your responsibility.

Further, while self-direction implies independence, it recognises limits in the interests of mutual support and cooperation with others.

If carried too far, commitment can become obsession. Don't get so involved with one or a few things that other areas of your life suffer. Avoid, for example, allowing work to stop you from enjoying any recreational activity, or recreation to leave no time for relationships.

Why self-direction and commitment are important to stress management

To avoid taking decisions or action creates tension and leaves problems unresolved. Decisiveness, action and persistence are needed to break unwanted patterns of behaviour and achieve personal change. A life of superficial involvement will lead to boredom and dissatisfaction.

Commitment is required for confidence to develop. You won't, for example, develop confidence in playing a musical instrument unless you commit yourself to practising with it.

Increased self-direction can lead to better health. Salvatore Maddi, from the University of Chicago, ran courses in self-management for men and women aimed at increasing their sense of personal control. These led to a reduction in anxiety, depression, obsessiveness, headaches, insomnia and blood pressure among his subjects, as well as more job satisfaction — benefits which lasted well beyond the end of each course.[7]

Aiming for your own goals rather than having others direct your life will affect how you implement many of the strategies in Part Three. It will determine how you manage your time, and help you assert yourself. By doing the things you want, you will also maintain more stimulation and variety in your life.

Developing self-direction and commitment

- Make a list of things you do that indicate lack of self-direction. Note behaviours such as asking for permission, avoiding doing something for fear of disapproval, unnecessarily seeking other people's opinions, and the like. Select one item each week and deliberately act differently in that respect, in line with how you would rather behave.

- Make a decision now to develop one new interest in which you will get absorbed. Commit yourself to taking steps toward it over the next week or so. See Chapter 15 for suggestions on this.
- Use *Rational Self-Analysis* (p. 80) and *imagery* (p. 86) to cope with any discomfort involved in carrying out these actions.

Flexibility

Flexible people can bend with the storm rather than be broken by it. They know how to *adapt* and adjust to new circumstances that call for fresh ways of thinking and behaving. They have *resilience* — the ability to bounce back from adversity.

The principle of flexibility

To be flexible is to be open to change in yourself and in the world. As circumstances alter, you are able to modify your plans and behaviour. You adopt new ways of thinking that help you cope with a changing world. You let others hold their own beliefs and do things in ways appropriate to them while doing what is right for you.

Flexibility in *thinking* means:

- Your values are preferences rather than rigid, unyielding rules.
- You are prepared to change your opinions in the light of new information and evidence.
- You view change as a challenge rather than a threat.

Flexibility in *behaviour* means:

- You are able to change direction when it is in your interests.
- You are willing to try new ways of dealing with problems and frustrations.
- You can let others do things their way.
- You avoid distressing yourself when others think or act in ways you dislike.

Why flexibility is important to stress management

Flexibility aids survival in a world that is forever changing, and in which the pace of change is increasing. A corresponding adjustment in attitudes and beliefs is required if distress is to be avoided. This is demonstrated continuously by the so-called generation gap. Parents who have become inflexible find it hard to cope when their children behave in ways unthinkable to them. People cope better when they see change as a *challenge* rather than a threat. As Suzanne Kubosa has found, this attitude is one of the characteristics of 'hardiness'.[8]

Flexibility makes for more effective problem-solving. As Roger Von Oech states, there are times when we need to step outside what we know or usually do and look at a problem from new angles in order to find a solution.[9] Even negative events — like being made redundant — can create opportunities to 'step outside'.

If you are flexible, you will find it easier to change your goals to suit altered circumstances. Growing older or sustaining a disability, for example, usually requires that one adapt to significant lifestyle changes.

Being flexible will help you break out of boring routines and maintain stimulation and variety in your life. It will also assist you to manage your time more effectively, by enabling you to change your plans to suit changing situations.

Developing flexibility

- Use *Rational Self-Analysis* (p. 80) to identify and change inflexible thinking. Note especially any demanding 'shoulds' or 'musts'.
- Expose yourself to new ways of looking at things. Read books that adopt positions different from yours, talk to people with opposing views, watch movies you would normally not bother with.
- Practise flexibility by rearranging your office or home furniture, hanging some new pictures or visiting places to which you have never been.
- Get into the habit of pausing before you take action on a problem and looking at alternative ways of solving it. In other words, attempt to act out of character on a regular basis.

Objective thinking

Flexibility and openness, as well as the other principles reviewed so far, require freedom from ways of thinking that are narrow-minded, sectarian, bigoted or fanatical, or that rely on uncritical acceptance of dogmatic beliefs or 'magical' explanations of the world and what happens in it.

Objective thinking is scientific in nature. There are four aspects to it — it is (1) empirical, (2) logical, (3) pragmatic, and (4) flexible.

Objective thinking is empirical

It is based on evidence gained from observation and experience rather than on subjective feelings or uncritical belief. It seeks to avoid distortions of reality — such as the seven common but self-defeating ways of thinking described on page 42 (originally outlined by Aaron Beck[10]).

Objective thinking is logical

It reaches conclusions that follow validly from the evidence. It is possible, as the example below demonstrates, to have the right *evidence* but draw the wrong *conclusions*:

Evidence: My supervisor has criticised me. I don't like being criticised.

Conclusion: I can't stand this. It shouldn't happen to me, and it shows that my supervisor's a rotten sod.

Even though the two pieces of evidence are correct, this does not make the conclusion correct also. The facts are that I have been criticised and I don't like this. However, 'I can't stand this', 'My supervisor's a rotten sod' and 'It shouldn't happen' are beliefs which go beyond the evidence and do not logically follow from it. More logical conclusions would be:

'My supervisor has done something I dislike.'
'This is unpleasant.'
'I'd prefer this not to happen to me.'

Illogical beliefs are often overgeneralisations. For example:

- Something that is *unpleasant* becomes *terrifying*. (Awfulising)
- Something that is *hard to bear*, becomes *intolerable*. (Discomfort intolerance)
- Because I *prefer* to avoid discomfort, I *absolutely must* avoid it. (Demanding)
- Because I *behaved* stupidly, I am *a stupid person*. (Self-rating)

To check the logic of your conclusions, ask yourself questions like:

- Do my conclusions truly follow from the evidence?
- What other conclusions may be possible?
- Am I catastrophising, demanding or self/other-rating?

Objective thinking is pragmatic

Science evaluates an idea not just on the basis of the evidence supporting it or its logical validity, but also on its usefulness to human beings. In other words, we need to be concerned with the effects, both short- and long-term, of what we believe. Questions to ask might be:

- What effect does believing this have on how I feel and behave?
- Does this belief help or hinder me in achieving my goals?

Objective thinking is flexible

To the objective thinker, nothing is absolute or the last word on a matter. Beliefs are theories that are subject to change as new evidence comes to hand and existing ideas are proved false. Objectivity encourages a continuing search for explanations that are more accurate and useful than the ones in current use.

Why objective thinking is important to stress management

Objective thinking is an essential component of any rational attitude or belief. For example, increasing your tolerance for frustration and discomfort means keeping their badness in perspective, rather than overstating them as 'awful' or 'intolerable'.

Unscientific thinking itself creates distress — for example, when people view criticism as unbearable, demand that they succeed, or rate their entire self when they have failed at something.

Believing you are controlled by outside forces, like fate or luck, can lead to feelings of anxiety, powerlessness and hopelessness, and cause you to take a passive approach to life and its problems.

Erroneous thinking, as we shall see later, also makes it hard to practise the coping strategies in Part Three.

Developing objective thinking

- Use *Rational Self-Analysis* (p. 80) to challenge erroneous thinking.
- Use *essays* (p. 84) to critically examine magical thinking.
- Read up on rational thinking.
- Developing other principles will also move you towards more objective ways of thinking (especially emotional and behavioural responsibility, self-direction, and flexibility).

Acceptance of reality

It makes sense, whenever possible, to change things you dislike. But there will always be some things you will not be able to change. You then have two choices: rail against fate and remain distressed; or accept reality and move on.

The principle of acceptance

To accept something is (1) to acknowledge it is a reality, (2) to believe there is no reason it 'should not' be, and (3) to see it as bearable. Consider these three aspects of acceptance in more detail:

1. *Acknowledging reality.* This involves admitting that reality — including unpleasant reality — is a fact. You see it as inevitable that many things will not be to your liking. You view uncertainty, frustration and disappointment as aspects of normal life.
2. *Believing there is no reason reality 'should not' be.* Although you may *prefer* that you, other people, things or circumstances be different from how they are (and perhaps even work at changing them), you avoid any *demand* that they not be as they are. You acknowledge there is no Law of the Universe which says they 'should' or 'must' be different.
3. *Accepting reality as bearable.* Some things you *dislike*, but you avoid catastrophising them into 'horrible' or 'unbearable'. You keep unwanted realities in perspective.

Acceptance of reality includes many things

There are countless realities people are called upon to accept. Here are some that are especially relevant to stress management:

- *Uncertainty.* In the real world there are no certainties. The outcomes of our actions can never be guaranteed. It is helpful to anticipate the future, but we can never know for sure what it holds.
- *Utopia is unlikely.* You and I will almost certainly never get everything we want. This includes total happiness or personal perfection. We will probably always experience some pain, anxiety or depression.
- *Limitations to personal change.* Many aspects of ourselves we can improve, such as the degree of anxiety or depression we experience. But there are some things that will not change no matter how much

we try, as Martin Seligman points out in his book *What You Can Change and What You Can't*.[11]

- *Changing others.* One thing we can never change is other people. Only they can change themselves. Accepting this reality can save a lot of pain for you and them.

What acceptance is not

Many people have trouble with the concept of acceptance. They think that to accept something means having to like it, agree with it, justify it, be indifferent to it or at least resign themselves to it.

Acceptance is none of these things. You can dislike something, consider it unjustified and prefer that it not be a fact. You can be concerned about it, and take action to change it if change is possible. But you can still accept it by rejecting any beliefs that it 'should not' be and that it absolutely 'must' be changed.

Why acceptance is important to stress management

Getting hot under the collar will not change something with which you are unhappy, and will only take up energy better used to confront the problem and do what you can about it. By reducing the intensity of your bad feelings, you will be less disabled by them. Paradoxically, acceptance will increase your chances of changing what you dislike!

Acceptance will help you tolerate what you cannot change, and allow you to avoid adding unnecessary emotional pain to an already unpleasant situation.

Finally, acceptance will help you avoid wasting time and energy and risking your emotional or physical health by striving for what is unattainable.

Developing acceptance of reality

- Note any demanding, non-accepting or catastrophising thoughts you have.
  - Believing that people or things 'should' be different from how they are; that it is 'awful' and 'intolerable' when things are not as they 'should' be; that the world 'should' be a fair place; that one 'should' always be treated fairly.
  - Feeling angry but unable to do anything about a situation.
  - 'Needing' to get other people to admit they are wrong because acceptance of a situation might mean giving away a sense of self-rightness.

- Keep reality in perspective. When facing an unpleasant development in your life:
  - Use the *time-projection* technique (p. 88).
  - Ask: 'Is this situation, event or possibility really so bad for me?'
  - Develop a *catastrophe scale* (p. 85).
  - Ask yourself: 'How much do I really need to upset myself over this?'
- Challenge any demands you make that reality not be as it is. Ask yourself:
  - 'Can I really change (this person, situation or development)?'
  - 'Though I would prefer things to be different from how they are, where is it written that they *should* be?'
  - 'Why *must* this not happen?'
  - 'Is demanding that this person change going to make them change? Or would I do better to try and understand how they see things and attempt to talk the matter over with them?'
- Practise acceptance:
  - Regularly remind yourself that human beings are fallible and not perfectible.
  - Don't retaliate when people do things you dislike.
  - See the world for what it really is (and always has been) — imperfect.
  - Practise being satisfied with compromises and less-than-perfect solutions to problems.

To sum up

We can sum up acceptance — and in fact all twelve rational principles — with a paraphrase of a well-known saying. To achieve happiness, there are three things for which to strive:

> *the courage to change the things we can*
> *the serenity to accept the things we can't*
> *and the wisdom to know the difference*[12]

One last thing. Don't let these principles become demands. They are ideals. Probably no-one could practise them all consistently. Rather than see them as absolute 'musts' for managing your stress, use them as *guidelines* to a better life.

Further reading on the Twelve Rational Principles

Self-knowledge

Asbell, Bernard. *What They Know About You*. Random House, New York, 1991.

McCutcheon, Marc. *The Compass in Your Nose and Other Astonishing Facts About Humans*. Schwartz and Wilkinson, Melbourne, 1989.

Self-acceptance and confidence

Dalrymple, Theodore. 'Letting the Steam out of Self-Esteem'. *Psychology Today*, 28:5, 24–6, 1995.

Hauck, P.A. *Overcoming the Rating Game: Beyond Self-love — Beyond Self-esteem*. Westminster/John Knox, Louisville, KY, 1992.

Enlightened self-interest

Selye, Hans. *Stress Without Distress*. Hodder & Stoughton, London, 1974.

Tolerance for frustration and discomfort

Dryden, Windy, and Gordon, Jack. *Beating the Comfort Trap*. Sheldon Press, London, 1993.

Hauck, Paul. *Overcoming Frustration and Anger*. The Westminster Press, Philadelphia, 1974.

Long-range enjoyment

Dryden, Windy, and Gordon, Jack. *Beating the Comfort Trap*. Sheldon Press, London, 1993.

Risk-taking

Roberts, Paul. 'Risk'. *Psychology Today*, 27:6 (Nov–Dec), 50–84, 1994.

Moderation

Birkedahl, Nonie. *The Habit Control Workbook*. New Harbinger Publications, Oakland, CA, 1990.

Kishline, Audrey. 'A Toast to Moderation'. *Psychology Today*, 29:1 (Jan–Feb), 53–6, 1996.

Emotional and behavioural responsibility

Bernard, Michael E. *Staying Rational in an Irrational World: Albert Ellis and Rational-Emotive Therapy*. Lyle Stuart, New York, 1986.

Ellis, Albert. *How to Stubbornly Refuse to Make Yourself Miserable About Anything*. Lyle Stuart, Secaucus, New Jersey, 1988.

The Twelve Rational Principles

Self-direction and commitment

Ellis, Albert, and Lange, Arthur. *How to Keep People from Pushing Your Buttons.* Citadel Press, New York, 1994.

Hauck, Paul. *How to Do What You Want to Do.* Sheldon Press, London, 1976.

Flexibility

Ingham, Christine. *Life Without Work: A time for change, growth and personal transformation.* HarperCollins Publishers, London, 1994.

Toffler, Alvin. *Powershift: Knowledge, wealth and violence at the edge of the 21st century.* Bantam Books, New York, 1990.

Von Oech, Roger. *A Whack on the Side of the Head.* Angus and Robertson Publishers, Sydney, 1984.

Objective thinking

Thouless, R.H. *Straight and Crooked Thinking.* Richard Clay, Suffolk, 1939.

Acceptance

Seligman, Martin E.P. *What You Can Change and What You Can't: The complete guide to successful self-improvement.* Random House, Sydney, 1994.

8
Rational Effectiveness Training

As we have seen, to turn distress into goodstress it is necessary to change dysfunctional ways of thinking. Rational Effectiveness Training (RET) provides a set of procedures for doing this.

RET has been developed by Dr Dominic DiMattia of the Albert Ellis Institute in New York. It is based on Rational-Emotive Behaviour Therapy, devised by Albert Ellis in the 1950s, and applies Dr Ellis' methods to stress management and coping effectiveness in a range of areas, including the workplace.[1]

How RET can help you

As the previous chapter has shown, to cope effectively with modern life, you need a rational philosophy for living. You also need to actually *live* according to that philosophy. New ways of feeling and behaving will not come automatically, but they will come with work and practice. Rational Effectiveness Training provides the tools to help you:

- Handle distressful emotional states.
- Change self-defeating behaviours.
- Eliminate the blocks to applying stress-management strategies.
- Increase your productivity.

A key RET technique: Rational Self-Analysis

Rational Self-Analysis (RSA) is a technique you can use to identify and change the thoughts involved when you experience distress or behave in self-defeating ways. Analysing your thinking will serve two useful purposes. It will help you reduce current distress and the likelihood of reacting the same way in future. Rational Self-Analysis uses the well-known *ABC* model developed by Albert Ellis.

How to complete a self-analysis

The first thing to do when you are feeling distressed or acting in a dysfunctional manner is to *stop*. Interrupt any self-defeating episodes or activity. Take time out to get your brain working on the problem. On a good-sized sheet of paper, follow this sequence:

1. Identify the *Activating event* — the stress trigger (*A*). What are you reacting to? Be brief — summarise only.
2. Identify the *Consequence* (*C*) — how you feel and are behaving in reaction to *A*.
3. Identify your *Beliefs* (*B*) — what you are telling yourself about *A*.
   - Look for any faulty *interpretations* (p. 42):
     – black-and-white thinking
     – filtering
     – overgeneralising
     – mind-reading
     – fortune-telling
     – emotional reasoning
     – personalising.
   - Even more important, identify your stress-inducing *evaluations* (p. 43). Ask questions like:
     – What is 'terrible'? (*awfulising*)
     – What is 'intolerable'? (*discomfort intolerance*)
     – What am I telling myself 'must'/'should' be (or not be)? (*demanding*)
     – What am I labelling myself (or others)? (*people-rating*).
   - Finally, identify the underlying *rule(s)* by which you are operating. Most rules will be variations of those listed on page 44.
4. Identify the new *Effect* you want (*E*). How would you prefer to feel or behave differently from *C*?
   - Your goal is to replace the self-defeating reaction with a more appropriate emotion or behaviour.
   - Make sure any new emotion you wish to feel is realistic. Rather than attempt to replace an intense negative emotion with a strongly positive one, aim to substitute a more moderate negative feeling. If you are anxious, for example, don't make your goal to 'feel great'. That would be unrealistic. You would do better aiming to 'be concerned'. This is still a negative emotion, but one more in proportion with *A* and less disabling than anxiety.

5. *Dispute* each of your beliefs (D). Substitute rational alternatives for those beliefs you decide are self-defeating. There are three ways to dispute a belief:
   - *Empirical* disputing:
     - 'Where is the proof?'
     - 'What evidence is there?'
     - 'Is there a law of nature that proves...?'
     - 'Or does the evidence really support some other conclusion?'
     - 'Is the 'law' really only in my head?'
   - *Logical* disputing:
     - 'Because (I want something/it's unpleasant/I made a mistake), does it follow logically that (I must get what I want/it's awful/I'm a total failure)?'
   - *Pragmatic* disputing:
     - 'Does it help?'
     - 'Does believing this enable me to be effective, achieve my goals and be happy?'
     - 'Or does it create unneeded distress, difficulties with other people, or barriers to achieving my goals?'
6. Finally, develop a plan for *Further action* (F). What can you do to reduce the chance of thinking and reacting the same old way in future? For ideas on self-help action assignments, see the following sections in this chapter on cognitive, imagery and behavioural techniques.

An example

Here is an example of a Rational Self-Analysis to show how it works in practice.

A. *Activating event (what started things off)*
  Head of Department criticised me in front of my team.
C. *Consequence (how I felt and/or behaved)*
  Stayed angry all day, took it out on my team, unable to concentrate on my work.
B. *Beliefs (what I told myself about A)*
  1. It was awful to be put down in front of my subordinates. (*awfulising*)
  2. I couldn't stand it. (*discomfort intolerance*)
  3. She should have talked to me in private. (*demanding*)
  4. She's a bitch. (*people-rating*)

5. I must always be treated in a fair and just manner, and it's awful and intolerable when I'm not. (*underlying rule*)
6. People should always do the right thing. When they don't, this shows how bad they are. (*underlying rule*)

E. *Effect I want (how I would prefer to feel/behave)*
   I would prefer to feel annoyed (rather than hostile), and assertively sort it out with her (rather than brood and take it out on others).

D. *Disputation and new beliefs (that will help me achieve the new Effect I want)*
   1. It was uncomfortable, but hardly terrifying!
   2. I didn't like it, but I stood it.
   3. It would certainly have been more thoughtful of her to talk to me in private; but where is it written that she 'should' behave correctly at all times?
   4. She isn't a 'bitch' — she's just a person who sometimes does bitchy things.
   5. I would always prefer to be treated fairly and justly, but nowhere is it written that I 'must'; and though I dislike poor treatment, I can survive it.
   6. It would be better if people always behaved correctly, but demanding that reality be other than it is will only screw me up. And a bad action does not make the total person bad.

F. *Further action (what I will do to avoid the same dysfunctional thinking and reactions in future)*
   1. Reread material on demanding and how I can combat it.
   2. Enrol for an assertiveness-training workshop.
   3. Once every day, deliberately choose to ignore a misdemeanour on the part of my staff or other people in my life to which I would normally react with distress.

Learning and using Rational Self-Analysis

The best way to learn Rational Self-Analysis is to practise it in writing. Eventually you will be able to do it in your head, although at times you will still find it helpful to get out pen and paper and follow a more formal procedure.

If you are like most people, you will start by doing analyses after episodes have occurred. Later, you will be able to do them while events are still happening. Eventually, you will begin to anticipate dysfunctional reactions and interrupt them at the start.

The technique of Rational Self-Analysis is described in more detail, along with some practice exercises, in my earlier book, *Choose to Be Happy*.[2]

Cognitive techniques

There are some additional tools that can help you deal with stress and develop a functional coping philosophy. Most of the techniques described in this and the next two sections can be used either alone or as part of a Rational Self-Analysis.

Reading

Keep educating yourself about the world and the people in it. Get information on particular problems from sources like books, magazine articles, pamphlets and the Internet.

Listening

- *Prerecorded self-help tapes*[3] have the advantage that you can listen to them while engaged in other activities like housework, driving, gardening or walking.
- *Record your own tapes.* Read into your tape recorder text from books or pamphlets you find helpful and would like to reuse.
- *Make tapes to help you cope with anxiety.* Record forceful, rational statements, then listen to them on a portable player while carrying out anxiety-provoking assignments.
- *Record a disputing sequence.* Conduct a debate in which you role-play both the self-defeating and rational parts of yourself. Make the rational part more forceful. You could have someone else listen to the tape to check how powerful and convincing your rational self is.

Writing

- *Diaries or logs.* Monitor self-defeating thoughts by keeping a diary of As, Bs and Cs for a week or two. Use this to check out your perceptions of reality (e.g. ask 'Am I *really* failing all the time?') or the extent of a problem on which you plan to work (e.g. ask 'How often do I overeat and under what circumstances?').
- *Essays.* Write an essay about one of your irrational beliefs, debating both sides of the issue. Or research and write up in detail a particular

problem area. Address questions like the following: What is known about the problem? What are the possible causes? What can be done about it? What blocks might get in the way of dealing with it? How can I overcome these?

- *Cards.* After disputing a self-defeating belief, take a small card and write the old belief on the top and the new belief at the bottom. Carry the card with you for a week or so, and take it out of your pocket or purse and read it eight to ten times a day. This will take less than thirty seconds each time, but the repetition can be a great aid in establishing a new rational belief. Don't be misled by the simplicity of this technique — it can be surprisingly effective. Note that a new thought requires daily practice or reinforcement for about twenty-one days before it becomes a habit, so refer to the card at least once a day for a few more weeks.

Miscellaneous cognitive techniques

- *Catastrophe scale.* This is a technique to get things back into perspective when you find yourself awfulising. On a sheet of paper draw a line down one side. Write *100%* at the top for absolutely catastrophic, *0%* at the bottom for OK (not a problem, neutral), and fill in the rest at 10% intervals. At each level, make a note of something you think could be fairly rated at that level. At *0%*, for example, you might write 'Having a quiet cup of coffee at home'; at *20%*, 'Having to mow the lawn when the rugby's on television'; at *70%*, 'Being burgled'; at *90%*, 'Being diagnosed with cancer'; at *100%*, 'Being burned alive' — and so on. Whenever you are upset about something, ascertain what rating you are subconsciously giving it and pencil that on your chart. Then see how it compares to the items already listed. You will probably realise you are exaggerating how bad it is, in which case move it down the list until you feel you have it in perspective. Keep the chart and add items to it from time to time.

- *Reframing.* This is another strategy for getting unpleasant events into perspective. One way to reframe them is to re-evaluate them as 'disappointing', 'concerning' or 'uncomfortable' rather than simply 'terrible' or 'dreadful'. Another way is to recognise that even the most negative experiences usually have a positive side to them, and to list all the positives you can think of. For example, redundancy entails not just loss of income, but also an opportunity to find a more satisfying job; criticism, unpleasant though it may feel at the time, can lead to personal growth.

- *Benefits calculation.* This is a way of breaking through decision-making blocks. It is based on the principle that we are likely to be happiest when our decisions take into account the desirability of both obtaining enjoyment now and continuing to get it in the future. To carry out a calculation, list all the factors that seem relevant to a decision. Note the likely short- and long-term consequences relating to each factor. Decide how much value or benefit each item has for you, be it positive or negative, then add up the figures, i.e. the pros and cons. A formal way to do a calculation is the 'four-window' decision-making method on page 216.

Imagery techniques

Rational emotive imagery (REI)

Drawing on the power of your imagination, REI can prepare you to deal with situations you would rather avoid because of the anxiety you feel about them. The steps, plus an example, are as follows:

Procedure	*Example*
1. Picture, vividly and clearly, the event or situation with which you are having trouble.	You have to inform a staff member their request for promotion has been turned down due to their poor performance record.
2. Allow yourself to feel — strongly — the self-defeating emotion which follows.	Anxiety.
3. Note the thoughts creating that emotion.	'He'll be upset.' 'I couldn't stand feeling responsible.' 'I must find a way to say it without upsetting him.'
4. Force the emotion to change to a more functional (though realistic) feeling. It is possible to do this, even if only briefly.	Concern.
5. Note the thoughts you used to change the emotion.	'It'll be unpleasant, but it won't kill me.' 'While I'd prefer him not to get upset, his emotions are his responsi-

bility.' 'I cannot control his feelings or be responsible for them.'

6. Practise the technique daily for a while.

Coping rehearsal

Coping rehearsal is a variation of REI. Imagine, first, experiencing the dysfunctional reaction you anticipate, then changing the self-defeating thinking involved, and feeling and behaving in more functional ways. Here are the steps to follow:

1. Do a Rational Self-Analysis.
2. Imagine yourself, as vividly as you can, in the situation you are concerned about, repeating the self-defeating beliefs you listed in the analysis.
3. Feel the emotions that follow, and see yourself behaving in the self-defeating ways you anticipate.
4. Imagine yourself, still in the situation, disputing and replacing the self-defeating beliefs, applying the rational alternatives you developed in the analysis. Feel your negative emotion reducing to a level you can handle, and visualise yourself acting appropriately.

You can use this to prepare yourself for many situations — behaving assertively, giving a talk, coping with a job interview, negotiating a contract, discussing a relationship problem, and so on.

The blow-up technique

Use the power of humour to get a feared situation into perspective. Imagine whatever it is you fear happening, then exaggerate it out of all proportion until you cannot help but be amused by it. Laughing at your fears will help you take control of them.

Say, for example, you are afraid to assert yourself with a coworker who dumps her work onto you. Visualise yourself telling her how you feel about it. See her accusing you loudly of being selfish and unwilling to work as part of a team, the rest of the office gathering around and agreeing with her, management being called in to deal with you, the police being summoned to take you away, your picture and a description of your actions broadcast on the television news, the country in uproar, the government passing an act to have you personally restrained from ever confronting anyone again, the army, complete with tanks and artillery, patrolling your workplace to make sure you stay in line.

Time projection

This technique is designed to show that one's life, and the world in general, carry on after a feared or unpleasant event has come and gone.

Visualise the event occurring, then imagine going forward in time a week, then a month, then six months, then a year, two years, and so on. Consider how you are likely to be feeling about the event at each of these points in time. You will eventually see that life will go on, even though you may need to make some adjustments.

You can use time projection to deal with a range of events and circumstances, such as actual or feared redundancy, loss of a contract, business failure, reduction in income, death of a loved one, disability, failure to pass an examination, and so on.

Behavioural techniques

It is important to put your cognitive changes into practice. Behavioural techniques, or 'action assignments', will help you in a number of ways. You can deepen and consolidate new, rational beliefs by acting in accordance with them and in opposition to the old, irrational ones. You can raise your tolerance for frustration and discomfort by deliberately exposing yourself to them. And you can experiment with and practise new ways of handling problematic situations.

Exposure

Exposure involves deliberately putting yourself into situations you tend to avoid. The main purposes of this are to test self-defeating beliefs and to increase your tolerance for discomfort.

It is a good idea to set up situations deliberately rather than wait for them to occur naturally. This allows you to prepare for them, so they are under your control. Real-life but managed practice of this kind will help you cope when events happen unexpectedly.

Here are some of the ways you can use exposure:

- *Shame-attacking*. This involves doing things you have previously avoided through fear of what other people might think. It will increase your tolerance for discomfort, reduce your overconcern about disapproval and increase your ability to take (sensible) risks. Your actions need to be such that other people are likely to notice and disapprove. For example:

- If you are obsessive about your appearance, leave home wearing non-matching items of clothing or without doing your usual grooming.
- If you worry about behaving correctly in front of others, break some minor social convention.
- Face any fear of appearing stupid by expressing an opinion to a group of people.

- *Risk-taking.* Challenge the belief that certain behaviours are too dangerous to risk when reason tells you that, while a favourable outcome cannot be guaranteed, they are worth the chance. For example:
  - Combat perfectionism or fear of failure by undertaking tasks at which you stand a good chance of failing or not matching your expectations.
  - Face fear of rejection by, say, talking to an attractive person at a party or asking someone to go out with you.

- *Desensitisation.* Deliberately enter situations you fear in order to demonstrate to yourself that you will at least survive them, if not learn to handle them. For example, if you are afraid of being in lifts, get into one several times a day for about a month or until such time as the fear diminishes.

Paradoxical behaviour

When you have difficulty with something, actually do it or make it happen. Behaving in new ways will help you change dysfunctional tendencies.

- *Act out of character.* If you are perfectionist, deliberately do some tasks to less than your usual standard. If you feel guilty because you think you are a 'selfish' person, treat yourself in some way each day for a week. If you tend to take life at a rush but worry you aren't getting enough done, deliberately slow down and take long breaks in which you do nothing but relax.

- *Postponing gratification.* If your problem is undue frustration when you have to wait for what you want, deliberately delay gratification in respect of one thing each day for a month or two.

Role-playing

Role-playing difficult situations will enable you to test out and practise different ways of coping with them before you face the real thing. Role-playing is often used when a situation involves communicating with others. Practising assertiveness is a common example.

Role-play with a trusted friend or colleague. Repeat the role-play until you feel you have got it right. Get the other person to give you feedback on how you came across so you can refine your technique.

Important points on using behavioural techniques

Don't take foolhardy risks. Avoid doing anything that might cause injury or unduly alarm or disrupt the lives of others.

The object of action assignments is not to 'succeed'. The real purpose is to expose yourself to problematic situations, either to test them out or to increase your tolerance. If your risk-taking was always a success, it would do little to raise your tolerance for discomfort. Often what you fear will not actually occur, but it is better that it sometimes does. For example, you could not develop the confidence to handle rejection if you had not been rejected a few times.

You can either start at the deep end and tackle the matters that bother you most, or take a graduated approach. With the latter, start by preparing a list of the things you find difficult, and order them according to the degree of anxiety you associate with each. Then confront these situations systematically, working your way up from the low-anxiety items to the high-anxiety ones. Don't be tempted to fudge the exercise by listing things that don't cause you some genuine discomfort. If you make it too easy, you will do little to increase your tolerance.

You can prepare yourself in advance of confronting a problematic situation by using any of the techniques described earlier. Imagery can help you cope emotionally. Role-playing can give you confidence.

For new behaviours to consolidate, you will usually need to perform them on a number of occasions over a period of time.

Making RET work for you

The importance of persevering

The techniques covered in this chapter will be very helpful as you seek to manage stress more effectively. But they will only work if you actually use them — and keep on using them. Bear in mind, too, that even though you may have been coping well for a while, humans tend to revert to previously dysfunctional methods of coping when under pressure. It is important, therefore, not to become discouraged when you find yourself worrying again, drinking more or avoiding discomfort like you used to. Use this as a signal that you are under extra stress and need to dust off your coping skills and make a fresh effort to put them into practice.

As time goes on, your improved ways of reacting will become more automatic, as you use slip-backs as opportunities to practise your coping skills, rather than view them as events that 'shouldn't' happen. Look on them as inevitable signs of human imperfection that you can use to your longer-term advantage.

Getting into action

Which of the techniques described in this chapter do you think will be most useful to you? List the top four:

1. _____
2. _____
3. _____
4. _____

Try one out today to see how it works. Then try each of the others over the next few weeks. Remember that you will probably need to use a technique more than once before it will work well for you. Perseverance is the key to success.

Further reading on Rational Effectiveness Training

DiMattia, Dominic. *Rational Effectiveness Training: Increasing personal productivity at work.* Institute for Rational-Emotive Therapy, New York, 1990.

Ellis, Albert. *Executive Leadership: A rational approach.* Institute for Rational Living, New York, 1972.

Part Three

Building on the Foundations — Practical
Skills for Coping with Life

Part Two laid down the foundations of effective stress management — the Twelve Rational Principles and the skills of Rational Effectiveness Training.

Part Three applies these using a number of specific strategies for coping with stress. Most of these strategies are typically taught on stress-management training courses, but, as we saw in Chapter 6, remain largely unused by many people. You will learn how to get round the blocks to their effective use by merging into them the principles and skills acquired in Part Two.

9
Have Clear and Realistic Goals

At the top of the list of strategies is goal-setting. This is because most of the others are based on the assumption that you know where you want to go with your life. Unfortunately, goal-setting is something to which many people pay only lip service. It is tempting to think: 'I know what I want. All I need to do is get on with it.' However, to avoid spending your life going down a succession of blind alleys, it is a wise idea to put some time into checking that what you think you want is what you really want. Explicit and challenging goals are necessary for three key reasons:

1. *Goals provide motivation.* You are only likely to feel motivated to do something, especially if it is less than pleasant, when you perceive that you have a good reason for doing it. The most common motivators are two sides of the same coin — human beings, when all is said and done, want (1) to feel good, and (2) to avoid pain. There are, though, many ways to feel good. You need to know which will work for you.

2. *Goals provide direction.* Goals help you direct your life, rather than simply react to other people, events and circumstances. They provide direction to your daily activities — knowing what your ultimate aims are will help you decide how to spend your days and hours. Goals also provide direction to other stress-management strategies. To manage your time effectively, for instance, you need to know what you want to achieve. Your goals will also guide your efforts to manage your financial resources, maintain a healthy level of stimulation, and solve problems.

3. *Goals provide a sense of accomplishment.* Your achievements will be most satisfying when you can see that they result from your own efforts to achieve a clearly defined objective. This in turn will create increased motivation to develop and aim for new goals.

Setting goals

Areas in which to set goals

There are many areas of life in which setting a direction can be important, including:

- personal development
- intellectual development
- spiritual development
- health
- relationships

- parenting
- work
- finance
- recreation

Goals, objectives and activities

Goals operate at more than one level:

1. *End goals* are what you want to achieve in the long term. They are sometimes referred to as *lifetime goals* or *ultimate goals*. They are general and abstract, the things to which you ultimately aspire, the end results you want. They may include personal, family, social, career, financial and community goals.
2. *Objectives* are more specific subgoals you aim for in the medium term, set up to help you move by stages toward your end goals — stepping stones along the way.
3. *Activities* are what you actually do to reach your objectives.

Most people will have a small number of end goals, more numerous objectives, and many activities. For each end goal there is usually more than one objective. In turn, for each objective there can be many activities. It may be easiest to visualise the relationship between these three types of goal as a series of branches from one level to the next (see p. 97).

An exercise to clarify your goals

The following exercise will help you clarify your end goals and objectives and develop some activities relevant to a high-priority aim. It is designed to draw on your gut feelings, so spend no more than a few minutes on each step. You can always go back later and revise your responses.

1. Write a list of your *end goals* (what you want to achieve in the long term). Be honest — don't censor any of your dreams.

2. Answer the question: 'How would I like to spend the next three years?' You may discover new end goals to add, and you may wish to turn some of those already listed into specific *objectives* (Check: 'Do these objectives help me move toward my end goals?').

3. Answer the question: 'If I knew I would be dead six months from today, how would I live until then?'

4. In the light of your answer to 3, do you want to revise your answers to 1 and 2?

5. Go through your list of end goals and prioritise them. Write *1* for the most important, *2* for the next, and so on.

6. Select one of the top-priority end goals you would like to focus on now, then look at the list of objectives you have developed at step 2. Pick out those that will help you to move toward the end goal and prioritise them.

7. Take objective no. 1 and list some activities that will help you achieve it. Be imaginative and write fast — brainstorm — and don't censor any ideas at this stage. Remember not to confuse goals or objectives with activities. A goal is something you want to achieve in the long run (e.g. keeping healthy). An objective is something you aim for in the medium term (e.g. achieving aerobic fitness). An activity is something you actually do (e.g. going for a jog each day).

8. Go back over your list of activities and cull the inappropriate or unworkable options. Order the remainder according to priority.

9. Select one top-priority activity you can action during the next week. Decide when you are going to do it.

Here are two examples to illustrate the process:

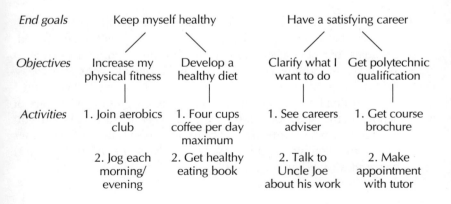

End goals	Keep myself healthy		Have a satisfying career	
Objectives	Increase my physical fitness	Develop a healthy diet	Clarify what I want to do	Get polytechnic qualification
Activities	1. Join aerobics club	1. Four cups coffee per day maximum	1. See careers adviser	1. Get course brochure
	2. Jog each morning/ evening	2. Get healthy eating book	2. Talk to Uncle Joe about his work	2. Make appointment with tutor

From time to time you will need to refine or modify your end goals, objectives and activities to suit changing circumstances and desires. You can carry out the above exercise time and again.

Tips for clarifying your end goals and objectives

A key question to ask yourself when defining your goals is: 'What do I really like and dislike?' As you consider this, keep in mind the following guidelines:

- *Be specific.* Vague goals provide little direction.
- *Write your goals down.* This will help you be specific, fix your goals in your mind, and enable you to review them from time to time.
- *Be honest with yourself.* If you want your goals to have motivating power, make sure they are what you really want.
- *Eliminate any 'shoulds'.* Your goals will only work for you when they reflect what you actually want rather than what you think you 'should' want.
- *Know what values are guiding your choice of goals.* Whereas goals are what we want to achieve, *values* are guidelines which affect both the goals we choose and how we go about achieving them. The Twelve Rational Principles described in Part Two contain values, e.g. *enlightened self-interest*, *long-range enjoyment* and *moderation*. It is important to be aware of the values which guide you. First, this allows you to check them out to ensure they are indeed yours, not someone else's, and are relevant to you at this time in your life. Second, you will be able to develop goals and objectives that are consistent with your values. Suggestions for clarifying your values follow in the next section.
- *Ensure your goals are achievable.* Unrealistic goals will not truly motivate you, because deep down you will know they cannot be reached. Set goals that can be achieved, albeit with time and hard work.
- *When you are unsure.* Some goals may be outside your awareness. Take note of your everyday actions and ask yourself: 'What am I really aiming for by doing this? What values are guiding my choice of actions in this situation?' You may need to get into action before you can identify what some of your goals are. Try out different activities to see what you like doing. This may involve some *risk-taking* (p.89) or *paradoxical behaviour* (p. 89).

Clarifying your values

The values we hold determine, largely, the goals we choose and what we do to pursue them. There are many values that people may embrace. Common ones are behaving honestly, telling the truth, preserving life, caring for others, keeping promises, being consistent, protecting the environment, and so forth. Your unique collection of values makes up your personal ideology or world view. If you are unsure of your own values, there are a number of things you can do to clarify them.

Observe your behaviour

Over a period of time, observe and record in a diary your responses — your desires and reactions — in a variety of situations. In each case, ask yourself what value(s) you think guided your responses. If you feel sad about somebody getting sick, for example, you may conclude that you value good health or the provision of effective preventative measures. Anger about a restrictive by-law may suggest you value personal freedom, or minimal intervention by external authority. Concern about an increase in burglaries may indicate security, or the sanctity of private property, is important to you. Feeling good about having a weekend free to spend with your children might indicate you place high value on family life.

Make a checklist

List all the headings you can think of under which your values might fall, then use these as prompts to fill in the actual values you hold in those areas. Typical headings might be:

- family
- recreation
- social life
- personal appearance
- ageing
- health
- relationships
- friends
- romance
- sex
- honesty
- spirituality
- education
- work
- art
- literature
- music
- finance
- material possessions
- politics
- the environment
- law and justice

Explore new values

Take opportunities to expose yourself to new values. Find out how other people see things. Read literature that will present you with new perspectives. Books on philosophy, for example, will provide new, alternative ways of viewing life.

Note that the Twelve Rational Principles represent a set of values. As you read about these, reflect on them, debate them with yourself or others and test them out, you will be introducing yourself to some new values.

Unlike when you were a child, when you accepted values uncritically, now you can scrutinise new and existing ideas using your adult intellect.

When values need changing

As you become more aware of your values, you may decide that some of them are less than desirable. Weigh them up and, if need be, change them.

How do you change a value? By using the procedures of Rational Effectiveness Training. A cognitive technique, such as *Rational Self-Analysis* (p. 80), will help you challenge an unhelpful value and develop a more functional alternative. Behavioural strategies like *exposure* (p. 88) or *acting out of character* (p. 89) will help consolidate new ways of thinking.

Overcoming the blocks to a goal-directed life

There can be many obstacles to effective goal-setting. Here are some of the more common, with rational principles that will help you overcome them:

Be aware of your values, and hold them as preferences

Being out of touch with your values will make it hard to set goals and make everyday decisions on what or what not to do. Perhaps you uncritically hold values you took on board as a child and have failed to check out as an adult. Whether or not you are aware of your values, if you see life in terms of 'shoulds' and 'musts', you are unlikely to set goals that are based on your real wants. You can help yourself in this area with the principles of *self-knowledge* (p. 54), *moderation* (p. 65) and *flexibility* (p. 71):

- Get in touch with what you really want, as opposed to what you 'should' want. If you discover that some of your desires are inappropriate — e.g. they aren't in your interests or are damaging to others — you can work at changing them. But your wants are the starting point for effective goal-setting.

- Avoid unrealistic goals, which set you up for failure, but extend yourself to your limits.
- Be guided by your goals and objectives — but not controlled by them. Adapt goals in response to changes in your environment, other people and yourself.

Confront anxiety and overcautiousness

Do you fear commitment? Are you unwilling to settle for one option and let go of others? Do you demand certainty and worry about making 'wrong' choices? Underlying these anxieties will be *ego anxiety* — fear of disapproval from others and of feeling bad about yourself — or *discomfort anxiety* — fear of frustration and discomfort. There are three rational principles that will help you here — *self-acceptance* (p. 55), *risk-taking* (p. 64) and *tolerance for frustration and discomfort* (p. 60):

- Remember that making mistakes does not mean you are 'useless' — all it demonstrates is that you are a person who sometimes makes mistakes. Failure to reach a goal or objective does not make *you* a failure.
- Accept that you may not reach some goals, or that your attempts may have undesirable consequences. But remind yourself that risk-taking is essential to forward movement.
- Rid yourself of the demand for certainty and accept that the only real guarantee in life is that there are no guarantees.
- Remind yourself that you will survive should you set goals which you ultimately fail to reach.
- See that giving up some options when you make a choice is at worst frustrating — not devastating.
- Accept that experiencing discomfort as you aim for your goals, and being frustrated when some are not achieved, are unavoidable realities of life; and that while you may *prefer* not to experience discomfort or frustration, there is no Law of the Universe that says these unpleasant emotions 'should' or 'must' not exist.

Be internally directed

If you believe your life is determined by outside forces, you will see little point in setting any direction for yourself. You can use three principles to overcome external directedness — *self-direction* (p. 68), *objective thinking* (p. 72) and *emotional and behavioural responsibility* (p. 66):

- Don't wait for others to direct your life for you.
- Assess the values you learned as a child and modify those that are not appropriate for you as an adult.
- Challenge any idea that the direction of your life is controlled by external forces, such as fate or luck, over which you have no influence.
- While you cannot have control over all that happens in your life, you do create your own reactions. Accordingly, remind yourself that you can survive emotionally even when your plans go awry.

Get rid of any 'unworthiness'

Do you believe you are too 'unworthy' or 'undeserving' to pursue your own goals, or that it is 'selfish' to do so? *Self-acceptance* (p. 55) and *enlightened self-interest* (p. 58) are the key principles here:

- Don't try to convince yourself that you are in fact 'worthy' (the conventional approach). Instead, get rid of any idea that you have to *be* deserving or worthy. Pursue your goals simply because you want to.
- Accept that while you dislike disapproval, what others may think of your goals or your attempts to reach them is less important than achieving a satisfying life.
- If being 'selfish' bothers you, remember that self-*interest* is part of being human and that you can practise it in an enlightened manner. Selfishness pays no heed to the wishes and concerns of others; self-interest takes these into account.

Have confidence in your own abilities

Do you have a low opinion of your own judgement? Do you doubt your ability to achieve your goals? Do you fear you would be unable to handle your emotions if things went badly? The principles of *self-knowledge* (p. 54), *risk-taking* (p. 64) and *confidence* (p. 55) are important here:

- Know where you lack experience and what your limits are, but keep this in perspective by acknowledging your assets as well.
- While keeping your goals realistic, be prepared to extend yourself and take some chances.
- Realise that while you don't have total control over your environment, you do have control over your internal reactions — so when things don't turn out as you'd like, you can still cope with your emotions.

Ensure your self-interest is balanced

Self-centredness ignores the reality that in addressing our own interests there are benefits that accrue from taking into account the interests of others. The principle of *enlightened self-interest* (p. 58) will help you do this:

- If you want to achieve satisfaction, ensure that your goals are truly your own, not someone else's.
- But keep in mind that you are more likely to achieve your goals if you take into account those of other people around you.

Consider both the short and the long term

Some people constantly pursue short-term gains to the detriment of longer-term possibilities. At the opposite extreme, others constantly strive toward long-term goals and rarely get to enjoy anything in the present. The principle of *long-range enjoyment* (p. 62) will help you get matters into perspective:

- You need two types of goals. Short-term goals bring early satisfaction; long-term goals involve work, patience and self-denial but provide greater rewards in the future. Keep the two in balance. (See *end goals*, *objectives* and *activities*, p. 96.)
- Invest your intellectual capital wisely. Don't squander your resources where they will have little effect in achieving your goals. Fight only the important battles — ignore the trivial ones. When, for example, the potential exists to get into conflict with others, ask yourself: 'Is this issue *really* important to me? Will fighting over it move me toward my goals? Or would I be better to let this one go and save my resources for the things that count?'

Be able to let go

Finally, appreciate that you cannot have everything. Use the principle of *acceptance of reality* (p. 75) to help yourself cope when a goal proves to be out of your reach. This will free you to get on with pursuing desirable alternatives.

Further reading on goals and values

Lakein, Alan. *How to Get Control of Your Time and Your Life*. Signet, New York, 1973.

10
Look After Your Body

Feeling good involves both mind and body. Each affects the other. You can create distress by abusing your body — or feel good by eating well, exercising and avoiding dangerous behaviour.

Are you stressing your body?

You may be creating distress through bad habits of nutrition and neglect, or exacerbating an already distressful situation by not taking care of your body.

How stress affects your body

When your body is reacting to stress, biochemical changes occur which have implications for your patterns of eating and exercising. For example:

- Distress causes the body's blood fat level to increase. If your diet includes a lot of fat, you can end up with an excessive level.
- Stress can cause dehydration. Tea, coffee and alcohol can make this worse because they are *diuretics* — they increase the rate of fluid loss.
- Prolonged stress uses up vitamins and minerals. You can anticipate this and at times of extra stress vary your diet or add supplements.
- When stressed, your immune system is less able to protect you against the bugs and chemicals to which you are exposed in day-to-day life. Lowered immunity can result both from common stressors like dietary deficiencies or excessive noise levels, and from major traumatic events such as bereavement or the break-up of a relationship.

When you are exposed to extra stress, you need to pay special attention to your diet. Unfortunately, many people under stress allow their dietary standards to fall — for instance, a grieving person may eat less than usual, or a coffee drinker increase their consumption.

How bad nutritional practice can create distress

- *Caffeine* stimulates production of adrenalin, which raises heart rate and blood pressure and irritates the lining of the stomach and intestines. Excess caffeine keeps the body's chemistry constantly 'on edge', making you more likely to react to things that happen around you, as well as causing headaches and sleep problems. As few as five caffeine drinks a day can produce these symptoms.
- *Nicotine* has a mixed effect. In the short term it may relax, but later it raises the heart rate. Its addictive nature also creates agitation when a cigarette isn't available. Nicotine is one of the most addictive substances known to humankind: it takes less than a second for the chemical to travel from the lung to the brain.
- *Sugar* can increase energy levels in the short term, but the boost is temporary because the body reacts by secreting insulin to hold down the amount of sugar in the bloodstream. Insulin tends to keep acting after it has normalised the blood-sugar level, causing a shortage of energy. A diet which includes an excessive intake of pure sugar raises insulin levels to the extent of causing fatigue, headaches, restlessness and difficulty thinking clearly.
- *Alcohol abuse* can lead to poor nutrition, liver damage, excess weight and the numerous social problems of addiction. It can cause low blood-sugar, increase blood pressure, damage the heart muscle and injure the stomach and gastrointestinal lining. Being a diuretic, it can compound the body's tendency to dehydrate when stressed.
- *Extreme dieting* places a lot of stress on the body. If you radically reduce your food intake, your body will automatically gear up to counter the threat to its equilibrium. It will slow down its functioning and burn calories at a lower rate to compensate for the shortage of fuel. The percentage of body fat will also increase, which means your body will need fewer calories than before you began the diet. If you return to a normal food intake, you will gain weight on fewer calories than before.

Good nutrition and exercise can help you manage stress

A diet that contains all the nutrients your body needs will defend you more effectively against distress. Under conditions of extra stress, such as work overload, bereavement, surgery or accident, a balanced diet will provide protection and aid recovery.

Exercise also helps in many ways. It elevates mood by increasing blood flow and releasing hormones which stimulate the brain and nervous system. It increases muscle functioning, improves oxygen delivery to the body, reduces blood pressure, and can improve the functioning of the immune system and help relieve headaches and asthma. It aids relaxation by decreasing tension in the muscles, and thus improves sleep. People who exercise regularly (and in moderation) are less likely to abuse substances or to use other unhealthy ways of coping with stress.

Eat to feel good

Good nutritional practices will help you avoid placing your body under unnecessary stress. We will start with the basics of everyday nutrition, then see how you can give your body some extra help at times of increased stress.

Maintain low-stress eating habits

- *Have regular, set meal times.* Avoid snatching meals on the run — allow enough time to eat without rushing. Make your meal times a priority. Don't eat a big meal late in the evening, otherwise your digestion will be working overtime when you are trying to sleep. Have breakfast every day — a lot of people skip what dietitians say is the most important meal of all. And, if it works for you, it is fine to eat a number of small meals through the day rather than the standard three big ones.
- *Don't eat more than you need.* Try to keep your body weight near its natural level.
- *Maintain a low fat intake.* Keep your total fat intake low, and as far as possible take it in polyunsaturated form (vegetable oils and some fish oils) rather than saturated (red meat, hard cheese, cream, eggs, butter, fried foods and many convenience foods).
- *Use sugar and salt sparingly.* Try to buy products without added sugar or salt. Minimise your consumption of convenience and takeaway foods, which often have high levels of sugar, fat and salt, as do luncheon meats and bacon.
- *Drink alcohol in moderation.* A standard drink is 200 ml of beer, a small glass of wine or one measure of spirits. Dietitians recommend that women keep their intake within fourteen drinks in any one week,

or three in any one session. For men, these totals are twenty-one and six respectively. Note that these levels are *maximums*, so you would be well advised to keep your normal intake considerably lower. The US Department of Health and Human Services defines moderate drinking as no more than one drink per day for women and two for men.[1] If you are driving, New Zealand Ministry of Health guidelines suggest no more than two drinks for women and three for men[2] (for some people these levels may need to be even lower). Drink slowly — one drink an hour is the limit your liver can process. Always eat when you drink — food delays the absorption of alcohol into the bloodstream.

- *Eat as much fibre as possible.* Sources include whole-grain bread, fibre-rich breakfast cereals and the skins of fruits and vegetables. Fibre helps to lower body cholesterol.
- *Drink a lot of water.* Water is the best fluid to drink during the day. It contains none of the sugars present in soft drinks and, to some extent, in fruit juice. You need about six to eight glasses of fluid each day, more when you exercise. Water helps fibre do its good work by bulking it out (which reduces the chance of constipation and bowel disorders), provides body cells with fluid and helps the kidneys flush out waste products.
- *Eat a lot of fruit and vegetables,* especially dark-green leafy vegetables. Obtain them as fresh as possible, eat them raw when you can, to cook them steam rather than boil, or boil only lightly. Fruit and vegetables contain antioxidants, which help the immune system.
- *Favour whole, unprocessed foods* — whole-grain bread and cereals, dried beans and peas, fresh fruit and vegetables, lean meat, poultry, seafood, non-fat or low-fat milk and cheeses.

Special nutrition for times of extra stress

When it is more stressed than usual, the body uses greater amounts of energy, drawn from the principal sources of protein, fat, carbohydrates and vitamins. You need to maintain your food intake and not fall into the common trap of eating less because your appetite has diminished.

- Maintain especially your intake of carbohydrate foods.
- Avoid foods high in salt — they will elevate your blood pressure.
- Keep up your intake of (1) vitamins — *C* (citrus fruits, berries, broccoli, tomatoes), *A* (silverbeet, broccoli, carrots, pumpkin, apricots)

and *E* (nuts, seeds, vegetable oils, whole-grain breads and cereals); and (2) minerals — calcium (silverbeet, broccoli, pumpkin, oranges), zinc and iron (red meat, dark poultry meat, dark-green leafy vegetables, dry beans and peas, whole grains, potatoes, dried fruit, berries, nuts).

- Keep your meals as regular as possible. Try to make meal times relaxing. If you have trouble eating large meals, it may help to eat a greater number of small meals and snacks.
- Don't attempt to diet at times of extra stress.

Getting dietary advice

The suggestions for good nutrition put forward in this chapter are of necessity very brief. You can get good detailed advice (and bad advice, too!) from numerous books on the subject. Look for those written by professionally qualified dietitians. If you have a computer and modem, you will find the Internet rich in free information on healthy eating. Should you have special needs, you may also benefit from consulting a professional; your doctor could refer you if necessary.

One final caution. If you are taking prescribed medication, or have any health problem that may preclude you from eating certain foods, check with your doctor before making any significant changes to your diet.

Exercise your body

Exercise, like healthy eating, can help you both avoid distress and cope better at times of extra stress.

Develop an exercise programme appropriate to you

Before starting an exercise regimen, it may be advisable to seek medical advice, especially if you are over thirty-five or have heart trouble, pains in the chest, dizzy spells, high blood pressure, or bone or joint problems.

To keep motivated, do exercise you find enjoyable. Consider what you prefer — competitive or non-competitive activities, exercising with others or on your own, exercise that requires a lot of concentration or only a little?

Develop a programme that is realistic given your circumstances, age and current level of fitness. Can you get outside, or do you need to exercise indoors?

There is one form of exercise most people are able to engage in — walking. This has many advantages over other kinds of exercise. It requires no specialised equipment, you don't have to dress up for it, you can wear a headset to play music or motivational tapes, and it gets you out of the house or office. You can increase the cardiovascular benefits by walking faster and swinging your arms.

There are two important types of exercise. *Aerobic* exercise is designed to keep the cardiovascular system fit. It needs to be intense enough to raise your heart rate for 20 minutes at least three times per week. You can achieve this through jogging, cycling, swimming or fast walking. *Flexing* exercises are designed to keep your body supple. The aim is to put each joint through its full range of movement at least once during the session. Stretching exercises are the most common. Design a programme that includes both *aerobic* and *flexing* exercise.

Start your programme gently. Straining your body could be dangerous, so don't push yourself or force your body to the point where it hurts. You will find yourself able to go further as your body becomes fitter and more supple. If you experience chest or muscular pain or any other distress, stop what you are doing and consult your doctor.

Exercise often — every second day at least. It is far better to exercise for 20 minutes each day than for 140 minutes once a week.

Keep up your exercise routine at times of extra stress

When life gets tough, we are often tempted to skip exercise — just when we need it more than ever. If you feel stressed, put your headset on and get walking. No time? Exercising will increase your efficiency, so the time spent on it may well be saved with interest.

Avoid dangerous behaviour

Dangerous chemicals

As well as avoiding overuse of nicotine and alcohol, take care with mood-altering drugs. Tranquillisers may bring short-term relief from tension, but at a longer-term cost of dependence and other problems. The dangers of illegal drugs such as marijuana, cocaine and LSD are well documented. Like tranquillisers, they may seductively offer short-term relief but at a longer-term cost.

Not all prescribed mood-altering drugs are problematic. Antidepressants, for example, if properly used can be a blessing for someone battling severe depression. It is extremely rare to become even psychologically addicted to antidepressants or experience long-term side effects. It is best to play it safe, however, by using drugs only with medical advice and supervision.

Extreme dieting

Radical dieting can severely stress the body. It is usually undertaken for the wrong reasons — as part of a health fad or an obsession with body image. Don't go on a special diet without consulting a qualified health professional. Check if you really do need the diet. If you do, find out the best way to go about it.

Overexercising

It is possible to get too much of a good thing. You can become addicted to your own adrenalin, or use exercise compulsively to avoid facing up to unhappiness in your life. The resulting overexertion can create its own distress. Fatigue can lead to sleep problems, anxiety and depression, and the time spent on obsessive exercise will disrupt other areas of your life.

If you find that exercise is becoming a compulsion and taking over, cut back. You will feel uncomfortable at first, but this will pass. Fill the time you save with other, more rewarding activities. If you cannot break the addiction alone, seek help.

A programme to change your self-care habits

1. *Start by assessing your problems.* Keep an 'eating and activity' log for about a week. Under 'day' and 'time', record your activities (eating/drinking/smoking/exercising), how much, where and with whom, and what you were feeling and thinking at the time. Evaluate what the diary shows, and plan any necessary corrective action.

Problems	*Solutions*
Excessive high-energy foods, e.g. takeaways, sweets, soft drinks.	Reduce to guidelines (p. 106).
Biscuits, sweets, desserts.	Eat foods like fruit or yoghurt instead.
Fat or oil.	Use other cooking methods like baking or microwaving.
Snacks during the day.	Avoid too much snacking — try drinking water or doing something physical.

Eating to improve mood/ emotional state.	Do something else to improve your mood when you feel bored or low: exercise, walk, talk to someone, read a book, get started on a task, dig the garden, etc.
Lack of exercise.	Look for opportunities to exercise — walk to the shops, use stairs rather than the lift.
TV snacking, tempted by rich foods at workplace cafeteria, etc.	Avoid situations that offer excessive temptation — take a cut lunch to work, decline invitations to eat out while building up your resistance. Enlist the support of people with whom you spend your meal times.
Excessive caffeine intake.	Limit coffee, tea, cocoa and some soft drinks to five cups a day (preferably three). Consider decaffeinated coffee or herbal tea as alternatives. Minimise food items and medications that contain caffeine, such as chocolate and cold remedies. Check labels on food and drink purchases.
Smoking.	Enrol in a cessation programme, see a counsellor or get a self-help book.
Excessive use of alcohol.	Reduce to guidelines (p. 106). If you need help, contact your medical adviser, a counsellor or an organisation like SMART Recovery.
Drug abuse.	Stop. If you need help, follow suggestions as for alcohol.

2. *Set your goals and objectives.* Specify your aims in terms of measurable behaviours, e.g. 'Eat breakfast every morning', 'Keep within three standard drinks of alcohol per day', 'Stop smoking by...', 'Eat fruit instead of sweets', 'Jog every second day'.
3. *Be clear about your reasons.* Write down the advantages of changing your behaviour so that when the going gets tough you can remind yourself why you are doing it.
4. *Identify and deal with any blocks.* Does your eating and activity log

reveal any potential blocks (see next section)? Design solutions, using the ideas in the previous three sections and the next.
5. *Develop a support system to help you change.* Enlist the aid of your partner, friends and anyone else you think could help.

Overcoming the blocks to healthy living

Don't let money get in the way
Do you see money — or, more precisely, the lack of it — as stopping you from eating well and following an exercise routine?

- Lack of finance may restrict your choices, but many forms of exercise cost relatively little or nothing at all, and it is possible to eat healthily on a limited budget. See Chapter 17 for ideas on making your money stretch further so you can achieve your goals.
- Note that healthy eating is cost-effective. Convenience foods are pricey, and ill health can be very expensive — consider not only doctors' bills but also the possibility of extended and possibly unpaid sick leave or early retirement due to poor health. The same is true of exercise. Walking, running and aerobic exercises at home are all free.

Get support
There may be a lack of support from those you live with for changing your eating patterns, and this will be especially difficult if you tend not to be assertive. Under such circumstances you will find it hard to get motivated to make changes on your own.

- Consider exercising with other people.
- If others know of your programme, this may increase your determination to see it through.
- Educate those you live with about why changing your diet is important.
- Keep changes sensible and avoid making demands of others. Don't, for example, insist that a big meat-eater become a total vegetarian. If you are the cook, do your best to make healthy meals that are well presented and interesting to eat.
- See Chapters 13 and 14 for more detailed guidance on obtaining support and cooperation from others.

Manage your time

Poor time management can lessen the time available for meal preparation and exercise.

- Note that there are two basic truths about any activity: (1) the only way to find the time to do something is to make it, and (2) what you spend your time on is almost always a matter of choice.
- Remember that a healthy body will help you concentrate better and be more efficient, so the time spent on self-care will almost certainly be cost-effective.
- See Chapter 16 for advice on managing time to achieve your goals.

Be able to accept yourself

Ego anxiety is a block to exercising for many people. Do you fear what others may think if you go out jogging or power-walking or appear at the gym in a leotard? Self-rating can lead to giving up — if you slip up in some way, e.g. by missing or not completing an exercise session, or eating a 'forbidden' food, you may tell yourself that you 'blew it' and are therefore obviously incapable so may as well give up completely.

Underlying such blocks will be rules like: 'I need love, respect and approval and must avoid disapproval from any source'; and 'To feel OK about myself I must achieve and succeed at whatever I do and make no mistakes.'

The rational principles that can help you here are *self-acceptance* (p. 55), *enlightened self-interest* (p. 58) and *acceptance of reality* (p. 75):

- Don't go on an extreme diet because of how you think you look.
- Avoid eating, drinking or using drugs out of fear others will put you down if you don't.
- Accept you may gain weight when you give up smoking and nicotine is no longer suppressing your appetite (or poisoning your body).
- Use *exposure* (p. 88) to help you with your fears of what others will think. Deliberately go power-walking or running at times and in places you know you will be seen. Wear your exercise gear when other people are around. Prepare yourself in advance with *imagery* (p. 86) or a rational belief *card* (p. 85).
- Expect to lapse on occasion. When you do, instead of condemning yourself as a hopeless case and giving up altogether, use it as an opportunity to learn and further develop your coping skills. Then get back to your self-help programme.

- Give your own health the priority it deserves — right towards the top of the list. But as you design and practise a more healthy lifestyle, keep in mind the wishes of others. Are you a care-giver who feels guilty about putting yourself first? Remember that your dependents will be better off in the long term if you look after yourself properly.
- Finally, accept that at age fifty you cannot be Miss World or Mr Universe — and that is OK.

Get motivated

Probably the most common reason people give up on exercise and healthy eating regimes is *low tolerance for frustration and discomfort*, based on beliefs and rules like the following:

Specific beliefs	*Underlying rules*
When I feel bad, I have to make myself feel better by (eating/smoking/drinking/etc.)	I can't stand physical or emotional discomfort and pain, so I must avoid them at all costs.
I can't stand how I feel when I go without (sugar/salt/a cigarette/etc.)	When I want something, I must have it.
It's too hard to (leave that cake alone/resist asking a colleague for a cigarette/etc.)	I can be happier by avoiding life's difficulties, unpleasantness and responsibilities, so must satisfy any desire I have.
Getting myself healthy should be easy and not require time and energy from me.	I must feel like doing something before I can do it.

You can overcome low tolerance by using the key principles of *tolerance for frustration and discomfort* (p. 60), *long-range enjoyment* (p. 62) and *self-knowledge* (p. 54), coupled with some Rational Effectiveness strategies (Chapter 8):

- Use rewards and punishments. If you slip up over one thing, deprive yourself of another — an enjoyable food, drink or activity, for example. When you achieve specific objectives, reward yourself. Don't carry punishment to extremes, and make it directly related to the omission concerned. Emphasise reward more than punishment.

Healthy eating and exercising will eventually become their own rewards; before long you won't want to miss your daily walk or eat fatty food. But while your body is adjusting, give your motivation all the help you can.

- Make it easier to resist temptation. Don't store unhealthy foods at home. Avoid shopping when you are hungry. Always have a shopping list and stick to it. Don't prepare more food than you need. Be clear about your rules: no snacking, trim the fat off meat, eat fruit instead of sweets, and so on. Do a *benefits calculation* (p. 86) on smoking, bingeing or other unhealthy behaviours.
- Expect to be uncomfortable as you change your eating patterns and get down to exercising. Anticipating discomfort makes it easier to cope with. Remind yourself that you will only come to like new food after you have eaten it for a while.
- Instead of overeating, drinking, smoking or using drugs to feel better, work at increasing your tolerance for bad feelings. Use *paradoxical behaviour* (p. 89). Make yourself do things you don't 'feel like' doing: resist the temptation to eat unhealthy foods until the desire is out of your system; persevere with healthy food until you come to like it; keep making yourself exercise until you begin to enjoy the exercise itself.
- Don't view the present discomfort of moderating your diet and increasing your exercise as just a pain. Look on it as helping you achieve long-term pleasure and enjoyment.
- To stay motivated, make sure you develop a diet or exercise regime that suits you. What happens to be trendy or to suit most people will not work for everyone. You may need to try out a variety of approaches before you discover what is best for you.

Three other rational principles can add to your motivation:

- *Emotional and behavioural responsibility* (p. 66). Don't blame others or the world at large for your state of health. Get moving and take change of it yourself.
- *Moderation* (p. 65). A radical 'all-or-nothing' approach to a new diet or exercise programme may cause you to give up because the improvement seems to be happening too slowly. Keep your expectations realistic; years of ingraining bad habits will not be undone in a few months.

- *Flexibility* (p. 71). Avoid *black-and-white thinking* (p. 42) over your diet or exercise routine. Don't make a pain out of what can be a pleasure. Allow yourself an indulgence now and then, without feeling guilty. Whenever you slip back, avoid the 'all-or-nothing' response; instead, pick yourself up, analyse the lessons and get back on track.

Further reading on healthy living

Consumers' Institute of New Zealand. *The Complete Exercise and Fitness Book.* CINZ, Wellington, 1985.

Goleman, Daniel, and Gurin, Joel (eds). *Mind/Body Medicine.* Consumer Reports Books, New York, 1993.

King, Olwyn. *Good For You: The latest word on what to eat.* Dietwise Publications, Petone, New Zealand, 1993.

Prussin, Rebecca, et al. *Hooked On Exercise: How to understand and manage exercise addiction.* Fireside/Parkside, New York, 1992.

Swarth, Judith. *Nutrition For Stress.* Foulshom and Co. Ltd, London, 1992.

11
Be Able to Relax Your Body and Mind

When the body gears up for action, the heart beats faster, breathing speeds up and the muscles tense. These reactions are designed to meet the *physical* demands of a situation — that is, either to fight off danger or to run from it.

Unfortunately, the body often gets it wrong. Most modern-day problems do not require a physical response. If a child is whining, you need to use your head, not your fists. Running away when the boss criticises you may say a lot for your physical fitness, but not much for your future as an executive.

Relaxation reduces arousal. When you relax, you slow things down and loosen up your muscles. Relaxation training can contribute to many aspects of daily life:

- anxiety control
- pain reduction
- coping with medical procedures
- lower blood pressure
- better sleep
- better functioning under pressure
- anger control
- increased confidence

Who will benefit?

You will probably benefit from relaxation training if you experience signs and symptoms like the following:

- *Symptoms:* muscle tension anywhere in the body; restlessness, a keyed-up feeling, easily startled; heart pounding, raised blood pressure; shortness of breath, increased breathing rate; headaches and migraines; trembling, nervous tics, grinding of the teeth; frequent need

117

to pass water, diarrhoea or constipation, indigestion, queasiness in the stomach; poor sleep.
- *Behaviours:* impatience, hyperactiveness, short temper; constantly busy to avoid feeling agitated; using tranquillisers or other drugs to calm yourself down.
- *Health problems:* hypertension, strokes, angina, heart attacks; chronic pain; stomach and duodenal ulcers; ulcerative colitis; irritable bowel syndrome; digestion problems; rheumatoid arthritis.

If you have a medical condition or mental-health problem, you will be wise to discuss relaxation with your health professional before proceeding with training. Go for a check-up if you have any of the following:

- *Medical conditions:* chest pains, hypertension, low blood pressure, cardiac disorder; asthma; diabetes; epilepsy; glaucoma; thyroid disorder; hypoglycaemia; narcolepsy; any disease of the gastrointestinal tract; recent surgery or injury; problems with your muscles.
- *Mental-health conditions:* It is not usually appropriate to do relaxation training when depressed because of the slowing down associated with depression. If a psychosis is present, consultation with an appropriate professional is essential.

Note that relaxation training will probably be ineffective if anxious *attitudes* are not first addressed. If your mind is actively worrying, this will undermine any attempt to relax your muscles. Use the techniques of Rational Effectiveness Training (Chapter 8) to reduce any worrying before you commence a relaxation programme.

The key principles of relaxation

Relaxation training will be more effective if you understand some basic principles.

- *Relaxation involves training.* It is not something a therapist does to you: it is something you learn to do yourself.
- *Learning involves practice.* Don't wait for a stressful situation to arise before you use your training. Practise so you are proficient *before* you need to apply it.
- *Relaxation is something you do.* You are not 'cured' when you have

completed the training. You need to consciously *apply* what you have learned when you feel stressed. True, the more you use it the more automatic it will become, but you will need to use it for some time before it starts to be habitual.

- *Relaxation training will focus on your muscles, breathing and mind.* Once you know how to make your muscles relax, regulate your breathing and focus your mind, you will be able to slow down both your physical and mental processes.
- *Relaxation is a way of taking control.* 'Letting go' of tension is the opposite of what your body is trying to do when stressed. There is a paradox here. By making your body 'let go' at your command, you are gaining greater control over it.

Three-stage relaxation training

Why bother with relaxation training? Why not just buy a relaxation tape and run it every time you feel uptight? Unfortunately, a lot of stress occurs in situations one cannot leave to play a tape. The boss is unlikely to adjourn a business meeting for half an hour so you can go away and put on your headset to calm down. Your kids probably won't stop demanding your attention while you pop into the lounge for twenty minutes to listen to dolphin sounds.

People in modern society need to be able to let go of their uptightness quickly, in the stressful situation itself, and when other people are around. The method outlined here combines several different approaches into a three-stage procedure for achieving this goal. The many hundreds of people to whom I have taught it have reported major alleviation of their stress symptoms. It is adapted from the method outlined by Goldfried and Davison.[1]

Introducing the three stages

Stage I is designed to help you make a clear distinction between tension and relaxation. Taking each of the main muscle groups in turn, you first tighten your muscles and concentrate on the exaggerated feeling of tension, then let go and focus on the contrasting sense of relaxation. This takes about thirty minutes. You practise once a day for seven to ten days. This will prepare you for Stage II.

Stage II is designed to relax the same muscle groups, but without tensing them first. This takes about fifteen minutes. You practise each day for seven to ten days. This will prepare you for the third and final stage.

Stage III is designed to show you how (1) to relax the whole body all at once, without using any exercises at all, and (2) to keep it relaxed even when you are carrying out day-to-day tasks. This takes about ten minutes. You practise for a few minutes each day for a month or so to consolidate the skill.

After following the method all the way through, you won't need to do the exercises again: you will know how to relax more or less instantly in any situation. It is then just a matter of frequently reminding yourself to use what you have learned.

Some important things to keep in mind

You are about to learn a new skill, like driving a car or playing a musical instrument. Don't expect to achieve deep levels of relaxation right away. As you practise, your results will steadily improve.

Adopt the attitude of 'going with' the process. You don't have to strive to relax: what you need to do is 'let it happen'.

If you have problems with your knees, back or any other joints, don't strain them when doing the exercises. If you wear contact lenses, take them out. When you tense a muscle group, you don't need to tense it as hard as you can — that can hurt. Just tense it to about three-quarters of the maximum possible tension.

When you let the tension go, release it instantly, and enjoy the sudden feeling of looseness.

Finally, do not attempt to use the training procedure while you are driving, operating machinery or in any other situation which requires alertness or concentration. Do your practice when you are alone, in a quiet place, with no responsibilities.

Getting started

The only material requirements are a high-backed chair with arms that fully supports your body, a quiet place in which to practise, and pencil and paper to record your progress. At each practice session, record the date, how tense you feel before you start and how tense you are after you have finished. Use this rating scale:

Completely relaxed					Moderate tension				Maximum tension	
0	10	20	30	40	50	60	70	80	90	100

Stage I

Draw up a form with headings as in the example below, then record the date and your current tension rating.

Date	Rating		Comments
	Before	After	e.g. interruptions, worrying, illness, headache,
			tiredness

When you are comfortably settled on your chair, check that you are breathing correctly. Place one hand on your abdomen, the other on your chest. Breathe in, taking the air deep into your body. The hand on your abdomen should rise, while the hand on your chest should stay still. Breath slowly, naturally and comfortably.

You are now ready to begin working on the main muscle groups of your body. Follow these steps for each group:

1. Tense the muscles.
2. Hold the tension for five seconds and concentrate on it.
3. Release the tension.
4. Concentrate on the feeling of relaxation for five seconds.
5. Repeat steps 1–4.
6. Check you are breathing properly, and wait another five seconds.
7. Move on to the next muscle group and repeat.

Working through all the main muscle groups of your body in this way will take about thirty minutes.

Start with the following sequence:

1. Clench your *left fist*. Hold it tight and feel the tension in your hand and forearm. Concentrate on the tension…(*5 second pause*)…
2. Now let go. Relax your left hand and let it rest on the arm of the chair. Let your fingers spread out, relaxed, and be aware of the difference between the tension you created before and the relaxation you can feel now…(*5 second pause*)…
3. Repeat steps 1 and 2.
4. Keep breathing deeply, taking the air right down into your abdomen. Breathing slowly, naturally and very comfortably…(*5 second pause*)…

Repeat this *tense – relax – tense – relax – check breathing* sequence with the following muscle groups:

1. Your *right hand*.
2. The *backs of your hands*. (Hold both hands in front of you and bend them back at the wrists so your fingers point toward the ceiling.)
3. Your *biceps*, the muscles in the upper arm. (Close your hands into fists, bend your elbows and bring your fists up toward your shoulders.)
4. Your *forehead*. (Wrinkle your forehead by raising your eyebrows as high as you can.)
5. Your *eyes*. (Close your eyes tightly, creating tension around them and in your cheeks.)
6. Your *jaws*. (Bite your teeth together hard.)
7. Your *mouth*. (Press your lips together hard, and at the same time press your tongue against the roof of your mouth.)
8. The *back of your neck*. (Press the back of your head against the chair, creating tension in the back of your neck and your upper back.)
9. The *front of your neck*. (Bend your head forward and press your chin into your chest, almost as hard as it will go.)
10. Your *shoulders*. (Shrug them as though you were trying to touch your ears.)
11. The muscles around your *shoulder blades*. (Push your shoulders back as though you were trying to touch them together.)
12. Your *back*. (Hold the top of your back against the chair and arch the middle right out, making your lower back quite hollow and creating tension all along your back.)
13. Your *chest*. (Take a deep breath, filling your lungs, and hold it.)
14. Your *stomach*. (Pull your stomach in, making it hard and tight.)
15. Your *bottom*. (Pull your buttocks together.)
16. Your *thighs* and *upper legs*. (Lift your feet off the floor, straighten your knees and point your toes away from you.)
17. Your *calves*. (Lift your feet off the floor, straighten your knees and point your toes back towards you.)

And now to finish…

1. Check back, one at a time, over the muscle groups you have just worked on. With each group, note whether any tension remains. If it does, focus on the muscles and direct them to relax, to loosen…(*5 second pause*)…
2. Relax the muscles in your feet, ankles and calves…(*5 second pause*)…shins, knees and thighs…(*5 second pause*)…buttocks and

hips...(*5 second pause*)...stomach, waist and lower back...(*5 second pause*)...upper back, chest and shoulders... (*5 second pause*)...upper arms, forearms and hands, through to your fingertips...(*5 second pause*)...throat and neck...(*5 second pause*)...jaw and eyes...(*5 second pause*)... Let all the muscles of your body relax, more and more, deeper and deeper...(*5 second pause*)...

3. Now sit quietly with your eyes closed, breathing deeply, slowly, naturally and comfortably. For a few minutes, do nothing more than that... (*2 minute pause*)...

4. Now consider your overall state of tension/relaxation. Decide approximately where you fall on the tension rating scale of 1–100.

5. Have a good stretch, and be fully alert.

6. Record your score on your record sheet.

From here on...

• Perform the same sequence each day for the next seven to ten days, or at least until you are scoring a relaxation level of 30 or below on two or three consecutive days.

• Remember this is only the first step in a three-stage training process. You will not be ready to apply your new relaxation skills in the outside world for a few weeks yet. Note, too, that at this stage the feeling of relaxation you create is unlikely to last for long after the practice session.

Stage II

Once you are used to identifying the difference between tension and relaxation, you are ready to move on. Stage II involves simply *letting go* each muscle group in turn, without first tensing. This will move you closer to the point where you can let your whole body relax instantly, without doing any exercises at all.

Start by recording your present tension level on a form like the one you prepared for Stage I. Then sit comfortably with all parts of your body supported so there is no need for any of your muscles to be tensed.

Now follow this sequence:

1. Breathe deeply, taking the air right down into your stomach. Breathing slowly, naturally and comfortably...(*3 second pause*)...

2. Direct your attention to your *right hand* and let go of any tensions there...(*3 second pause*)... Relax the muscles in your right hand as far

as you are able…(*3 second pause*)… Let go further and further…
(*3 second pause*)…

Repeat this *breathing – relax – relax* sequence with the following muscle groups:

1. Your *right forearm*.
2. Your *upper right arm*.
3. Your *left hand*.
4. Your *left forearm*.
5. Your *upper left arm*.
6. Your *shoulders*.
7. Your *forehead*.
8. Your *eyes*.
9. Your *cheeks*.
10. Your *jaws*.
11. Your *neck*.
12. Your *chest*.
13. Your *stomach*.
14. Your *hips and buttocks*.
15. Your *thighs*.
16. Your *calves*.
17. Your *feet*.

To finish…

1. Even when you are feeling very relaxed, it is often possible to let go just a little bit more. To do this, count from 1 to 10, repeating the following words (or something like them) with each number. At each step, let go a little bit more than before.
2. One, 'Relax, just relax…' (*3 second pause*)… Two, 'Deeper and deeper, further and further relaxed…' (*3 second pause*)… Three, 'Letting go, more and more, deeper and deeper…' (*3 second pause*)… Four, 'Getting heavier and looser, more and more relaxed…' (*3 second pause*)… Five, 'Further and further relaxed…' (*3 second pause*)… Six, 'More and more, further and further…' (*3 second pause*)… Seven, 'Deeper and deeper, more and more relaxed…' (*3 second pause*)… Eight, 'Letting go more and more…' (*3 second pause*)… Nine, 'My whole body more and more relaxed, deeper and deeper…' (*3 second pause*)… And ten, 'Just continuing to relax, more and more, further and further relaxed…' (*3 second pause*)…

3. If you are now at 30 or below on your tension rating scale — that is, feeling quite relaxed — you can try an exercise that will help you relax even more. Focus your attention on the point at which your breath leaves your body, and allow your body to relax a little more each time you breathe out. This will help you clear and relax your mind, as well as increase the relaxation in your body. Do this now, for a few minutes…(*3 minute pause*)…

4. Now consider your overall state of tension/relaxation. Decide approximately where you fall on the tension rating scale of 0–100.

5. Have a good stretch, and be fully alert.

6. Record your score on your record sheet.

From here on…

• Practise this stage each day until you are regularly achieving a relaxation level of 30 or below (for five to seven days in a row).

Stage III

After adequate practice on Stage II, you are ready to learn how to relax your entire body inconspicuously and quickly in just about any situation, even while carrying out tasks and activities or in the presence of other people.

Your aim with Stage III is to learn how to be aware of any unnecessary tension that creeps in, and to quickly let it go, in a selective fashion, depending on what the situation requires of your muscles.

Follow this sequence:

1. Relax in your chair for five to ten minutes, or until you have achieved a relaxation level of 30 or below.

2. You need *some* tension in *some* parts of your body to carry out day-to-day activities. However, other parts of the body may not need to be tensed, and it is this unneeded tension that is now to be your focus.

3. Fix your gaze on some object on the wall, such as a picture or light switch. Notice that to do this you need to slightly tense your neck (to keep your head upright) and your eyes (to keep them open and focused). However, identify any *other* tension that has crept in (e.g. in your arms, legs, stomach, etc.) and let it go while still focusing on the object.

4. Repeat step 3 with a number of more demanding tasks. For example, hold a book in your hands and turn it over and over, or stand up and

look out of a window. With each task, identify which muscles need to be tensed to carry it out, then be aware of and get rid of any unneeded tension that creeps into other parts of your body. Continue the task for several minutes, until you can remain tension free while carrying it out.

From here on…

• Practise the Stage III exercise for a few minutes each day for several months. This will help you consolidate the relaxation habit.

Using a tape recorder

An alternative way to learn the three-stage relaxation procedure is to tape-record the instructions for Stages I and II. Then all you have to do is follow the tape whenever you practise. You can record the instructions yourself or ask someone else to do it for you. Speak in a slow, measured, calm manner.

An additional technique

Once you have completed the three-stage training, you will be able to relax quickly and efficiently in just about any situation. Over time, you can add further techniques. One that is particularly useful I call the *breathing-focus* technique.

This procedure is good for clearing the mind when it is overactive or you are worrying and unable to relax. It can also help you get to sleep, and you can use it for five minutes or so to refresh body and mind during the day. It is one of the simplest and most useful techniques I teach my clients. You have already used it to some degree if you have completed Stage II of the three-stage method.

The technique

1. Sit (or lie) in a comfortable position.
2. Breathe in slowly and deeply. Take a good, deep breath right down into your abdomen, filling yourself with health-giving oxygen.
3. Hold your breath for about one second.
4. Slowly breathe out. As you do, focus on your breath as it leaves your body. Focus on the centre of your face, visualising the breath leaving through your nose and/or mouth.
5. Each time you breathe out, imagine that a little more of the tension leaves your body along with your breath. Let your body, from the top of

your head to the tips of your fingers and down to your feet, slump a little more each time you breathe out. Breathe right out, expelling all the old air and waste products.

6. Pause for about a second before breathing in again.

Some tips

To make the procedure more effective:

- Maintain your focus on the centre of your face, where the breath enters and leaves your body. If your attention wanders, bring it back. Holding the one point of focus will keep your mind from drifting back to stressful thoughts.
- When thoughts intrude, allow them to pass by and return to focusing on your breathing.
- Whenever you become aware of noises around you, instead of trying to shut them out, focus on them briefly. Treat noise as a natural part of your environment rather than something to be avoided. Some people find it helpful to think of themselves as 'merging' with the noise, or 'absorbing' it. This strategy can be surprisingly effective when you are trying to work, relax or sleep in a noisy situation.
- Don't become obsessive about getting your breathing 'perfect'. Don't force yourself to breathe deeply. Adopt the attitude of 'allowing' it to happen.

When to use it

- Use the breathing-focus technique whenever you feel stressed, especially when stressful thoughts keep intruding.
- Use it to get to sleep when your mind is overactive or your body is tense.
- Try using it routinely for five or ten minutes one or more times a day. This will increase your alertness and concentration, and also act as a stress preventative.

I perform this exercise every day, at least once (at midday), often at several different times. I have a cheap kitchen timer which I set for a maximum of ten minutes to ensure I don't drift off to sleep. This sets me up to be relaxed but alert, especially in the afternoon, when my energy and concentration tend to be at a low ebb.

Making relaxation work in everyday life

Remember that the relaxation skills you learn are just that — skills. They are not a cure. You will benefit from what you learn in proportion to the extent you apply it. Get into the habit of stopping at regular intervals throughout the day to consider: 'Am I tense or relaxed right now? Could I be more relaxed than I am?'

Develop a reminder system. Get some coloured stickers (dots or stars) and place them where you will see them through the day — on the bathroom mirror, above the kitchen sink, on the car speedometer, on your watchstrap, briefcase, purse or wallet.

Finally, keep in mind that relaxation training is not a total solution to stress. Don't neglect the self-defeating attitudes and beliefs that create stress in the first place, and which can stop you applying your new-found relaxation skills.

Overcoming the blocks to relaxation

Lack of time

Probably the most common block to learning and using relaxation techniques is the 'I don't have time' argument. Use the principle of *long-range enjoyment* (p. 62) to help yourself here:

- Note that being able to relax your body and mind will be cost effective. It will reduce your fatigue, increase your alertness and concentration, and increase your efficiency and productivity.
- Taking the time to learn and use relaxation techniques, instead of resorting to quick fixes like tranquillisers, alcohol or marijuana, will help you control stress much better in the long run.
- If you do have significant trouble with time, see Chapter 16.

When relaxation doesn't seem to work

If relaxation doesn't seem to work for you, it may be that (1) you are not a suitable candidate for relaxation training, (2) your mind is very active, perhaps through worry, while you are trying to relax, or (3) you haven't really practised the three-stage relaxation method faithfully. Relevant principles here are *self-knowledge* (p. 54) and *self-direction* (p. 68):

- See the suitability criteria on pages 117–18.

- Experiment. If none of the suggestions in this chapter sits well with you, check out alternative strategies such as meditation, visualisation or biofeedback. (Your doctor, local mental health service or other health professional may be able to advise you where to get information.) Use relaxation strategies that work for you, no matter what your family, friends or colleagues say you 'should' do.
- Do some work on your tendency to worry before attempting further relaxation training. Regular use of *Rational Self-Analysis* (p. 80) is an excellent tool for chipping away at an undesirable habit.
- Make sure you have taken the time to follow the three-stage method correctly, especially the daily practice.

Do you become panicky?

A small proportion of people who begin relaxation training become more anxious, and possibly even panicky, when they have started to relax. This is usually due to a sense of losing control as they begin to let go. Applying the principle of *tolerance for discomfort* (p. 60) is helpful:

- Remind yourself that anxiety is unpleasant but not 'horrific', uncomfortable but not 'unbearable'. Persevere through the discomfort — the sensation will pass.
- If you feel afraid when you close your eyes during relaxation training, keep them open to begin with.
- Most importantly, use *Rational Self-Analysis* (p. 80) to uncover and deal with the thoughts creating your anxiety.

A final note

Emotional and behavioural responsibility (p. 66) is another key principle you can use to make relaxation work for you:

- Don't blame others for the way you feel — that will stop you taking charge.
- Don't rely on professionals to fix your tension. You can get advice and help, but in the end only you can put the advice into practice.
- Taking responsibility will almost certainly make relaxation a useful tool you can use in many areas of your life.

Further reading on relaxation

Davis, Martha, et al. *The Relaxation and Stress Reduction Workbook*. New Harbinger Publications, Oakland, CA, 1988.

Fried, Robert. *The Breath Connection: How to reduce psychosomatic and stress-related disorders with easy-to-do breathing exercises*. Plenum, NY, 1990.

Goleman, Daniel, and Gurin, Joel (eds). *Mind/Body Medicine*. Consumer Reports Books, New York, 1993.

Obtaining a relaxation tape

A professionally prepared recording of the *three-stage method*, with the *breathing-focus* technique included, is available for purchase. The best way to obtain the cassette and instruction booklet package is to use the Internet (http://www.voyager.co.nz/~rational/public/resources.htm).

12
Sleep Well

Feeling tired occasionally during the day is normal for most people. But if you feel tired frequently or constantly, you may become irritable and short-tempered. You will find it hard to carry out even routine tasks. Your concentration, spontaneity and creativity will be affected. Chronic tiredness increases the likelihood of accidents and makes a person more vulnerable to depression and anxiety.

The sleep questionnaire

Do you have trouble sleeping? If so, the questionnaire which follows will help you identify the causes. Tick any boxes that apply to you.

Sleep environment

☐ Noise
☐ Shift-work
☐ Time-zone changes
☐ Bed partner restless or noisy or snores
☐ Other _____

☐ Too cool
☐ Too warm
☐ Uncomfortable bed

Sleep routine

☐ Heavy meal close to bedtime
☐ Little exercise during the day
☐ Exercise close to bedtime
☐ Work in bed or in your bedroom
☐ Hard to switch off your mind when you go to bed
☐ Irregular bed- and getting-up times
☐ Other _____

☐ Read or watch television in bed
☐ Tense while lying in bed
☐ Uncomfortable bed

Substance use

- ☐ Prescribed sleeping pills
- ☐ Over-the-counter sleep aids
- ☐ Tranquillisers
- ☐ Diuretic or water-reducing medication

- ☐ Cold remedies
- ☐ Appetite suppressants
- ☐ Stimulants
- ☐ Slimming pills

- ☐ Caffeine: ___ cups of tea, coffee or other caffeinated drinks per day, last cup at ____ p.m.
- ☐ Other fluids: ___ cups/glasses in evening, last at ____ p.m.
- ☐ Chocolate: _____ during the day, last at ____ p.m.
- ☐ Alcohol: _____ standard drinks per day, last drink at ____ p.m.
  (standard drink = 200 ml beer, small glass wine, one measure spirits)
- ☐ Nicotine: ____ cigarettes/cigars/pipes per day.
- ☐ Drugs such as heroin, cocaine, cannabis, amphetamines, LSD or other hallucinogens.

Emotions

- ☐ Anxiety/worry
- ☐ Panic attacks
- ☐ Anger
- ☐ Other _____

- ☐ Depression
- ☐ Stress
- ☐ Guilt

Physical health

- ☐ Pain
- ☐ Heart problems
- ☐ Breathing problems
- ☐ Emphysema
- ☐ Asthma
- ☐ Hiatus hernia
- ☐ Enlarged prostate
- ☐ Stomach and digestive disorders
- ☐ High blood pressure
- ☐ Other _____

- ☐ Cancer
- ☐ Kidney failure
- ☐ Parkinson's disease
- ☐ Starvation (including anorexia)
- ☐ Food allergies
- ☐ Significantly over- or underweight
- ☐ Cough
- ☐ Toothache
- ☐ Arthritis

Miscellaneous symptoms

☐ You wake in the early-morning hours and cannot get back to sleep, no matter what you do.

☐ You fall asleep uncontrollably at odd times during the day, either for a few seconds or for longer periods.

☐ After experiencing a strong emotion (such as hilarity, anger or surprise) your muscles feel weak.

☐ Just before going to sleep and just after you wake you are unable to move or speak.

☐ At the moment you are falling asleep or waking up you experience vivid, dreamlike images.

☐ You have a restless, uncomfortable feeling in your legs that you can relieve only by moving or stimulating them, e.g. by walking around.

While asleep, you experience:

☐ Frequent leg or arm jerks, or general thrashing around
☐ Snoring
☐ Irregular breathing or gasping for breath
☐ Intense anxiety (not associated with any dream) which leads you to cry out (as an adult).
☐ Sleepwalking (as an adult).

Beliefs about sleep

Listed below are a number of statements reflecting beliefs and attitudes concerning sleep. Indicate to what extent you personally agree or disagree with each, using this scale.

Strongly disagree	Disagree	Unsure	Agree	Strongly agree
1	2	3	4	5

__ Going for one or two nights without sleep will inevitably have serious consequences.

__ Chronic insomnia will lead to a nervous breakdown.

__ If I spend more time in bed, I can get more sleep and feel better the next day.

__ When it's hard to sleep, the best thing is to stay in bed and keep trying.

__ If I have a poor night's sleep, I won't be able to function the next day.

__ It's better to take a sleeping pill than have a poor night's sleep.

__ There's nothing wrong with using sleeping pills on a permanent basis.

__ Everyone needs eight hours of sleep.

__ Insomnia is the result of ageing and there isn't much that can be done about it.

__ Feeling bad or functioning poorly is mostly caused by not sleeping well.

__ Insomnia is mainly caused by biochemical factors in the body.

__ Alcohol before bedtime is a good way to get a night's sleep.

__ I must be able to feel and function at my best every day, which requires a good night's sleep.

__ There's little I can do to handle the tiredness, irritability, anxiety and poor functioning that results from poor sleep.

__ It's awful to have a sleepless night and I can't stand the way I feel the next day.

__ I absolutely must get a good sleep every night.

__ I should be able to sleep well every night, no matter where I am or what's happening in my life.

__ Insomnia is ruining my ability to enjoy life and stopping me from achieving my goals.

Analysing your answers

The items you ticked in the questionnaire will help you identify problem areas to work on. Solutions are presented in various parts of this chapter.

- *Substances.* If you ticked any of the medications, see your doctor. Other items in this section require that you either modify your intake or give up entirely. Be wary of any consumption of caffeine within six hours of bedtime, or more than one standard drink of alcohol after your evening meal (see pp. 106–7). (Note, though, that caffeine and alcohol at night do not affect everyone the same way, so you may need to experiment.)

- *Emotions.* Deal with any that you ticked, using the strategies of *Rational Effectiveness Training* (Chapter 8), or seek professional help if necessary.

- *Physical health.* Seek appropriate medical advice for any problems in this section.

- *Miscellaneous.* The items listed all warrant seeking medical advice. Snoring, for example, inhibits the brain from entering a key phase of sleep and reduces the body's oxygen levels at night. The poor-quality sleep which results leads to daytime drowsiness. Heavy snorers may benefit from seeing an ear, nose and throat specialist as medical procedures are now available to correct the abnormalities that cause snoring.

- *Beliefs.* Look at any items in this section for which you gave yourself a score of 4 or 5. All the statements listed are either myths or irrational beliefs about sleeping.
  - You may have noticed that worrying about sleeplessness causes it! A vicious circle is set up. Demanding that you sleep will keep you awake. Getting to sleep involves 'letting go', so 'trying' makes it less likely you will drop off. 'I *need* eight hours sleep' leads to anxiety, anxiety leads to sleeplessness, and so it goes round.
  - Exaggerating and awfulising can create self-fulfilling prophecies. If you tell yourself you are going to have a bad day, you are likely to make yourself have one.
  - Many people make the assumption that disturbed sleep is inevitable with increasing age. Some older people may find it harder to sleep because of reduced melatonin levels; however, research shows that appropriate treatment can usually help older people sleep well.[1]
  - At the end of this chapter is a further list of self-defeating beliefs about sleep, with a rational alternative for each.

Some facts about sleep

Most people seem to benefit from between six and ten hours' sleep a night, with the average being about seven and a half. As you get older, your sleep requirements may reduce. What matters is not how many hours you spend in bed but how you feel in the morning.

It is possible to catch up on lost sleep. If you miss a night or even two, one good night's rest will usually be enough to make up the deficit.

There are a number of stages to one's sleep during the night. Each of these is important, and probably serves a specific function in restoring the body and mind. For example, the stage known as rapid eye movement (REM) sleep (so-called because during it the eyes move rapidly under their lids) is associated with dreaming and an accelerated flow of blood through the brain. One theory has it that this process restores the brain. The other main stage of sleep — non-REM, or quiet, sleep — may serve to restore the body. All the stages of sleep are important.

The basics of sleeping well

The first step to resolving a sleep problem is to ensure you are observing some basic, day-to-day routines that are important to good sleep (referred to in the professional literature as 'sleep hygiene'). Later we shall look at some specific solutions to particular sleep problems.

What you do while awake affects how you sleep

- *Keep daytime stress under control.* Use the strategies in this book to alleviate the things you worry about, manage your time effectively, take regular exercise, develop creative hobbies and deal with emotions like anger and anxiety.
- *Practise good eating habits.* Eat sleep-enhancing foods such as milk, eggs, meat, nuts, fish, cheese and soybeans. Have at least one hot meal each day, and eat in a relaxed manner, sitting down, at regular times. Avoid a heavy meal close to bedtime.
- *Exercise regularly during the day.* But see the comments below on exercise in the evening.
- *Is it wise to nap during the day?* For some people, daytime napping makes it hard to sleep at night. For others, napping helps them sleep better (as well as refreshing them during the day). You need to experiment. The *breathing-focus* relaxation technique (p. 126) is one way to refresh yourself during the day without going to sleep.

Ensure your environment is conducive to sleep

Is your bed comfortable? Keep your bedroom at a moderate temperature — not too warm, not too cool. Make your bedroom reasonably dark, but with provision for light to get in when morning comes. Dark and light are perceived by the brain as cues for the body system to put itself to sleep and wake up.

Have regular sleeping hours

You will sleep better if your system becomes used to a regular routine.

- *Retire and get up at roughly the same time* each night and morning. Sleeping in is not a good idea. Maintain your routine to within an hour every day.
- *Resist the temptation to stay in bed* when you are not fully asleep.

Dozing in the morning, for instance, will make it harder to get a deep sleep the following night.

Develop a good pre-bedtime routine

- *Things to avoid close to bedtime* include vigorous exercise (this will stimulate you when you need to be winding down), falling asleep in front of the television, consumption of caffeine or alcohol, smoking, eating chocolate and some cheeses. Not everyone is affected in the same way or to the same degree by these; experiment to see what makes a difference to you.
- *Prepare yourself physically.* Try to be more physically than mentally tired at bedtime. Take a light walk, then a warm bath. Have a sleep-inducing supper of foods such as cereal with milk or bread and honey, and a warm milk drink or herb tea.
- *Prepare yourself mentally.* Avoid dwelling on stressful matters that cannot be resolved before bedtime: arguments, unhappy thoughts, anger, unsolved problems. To shed any excitement, engage in winding-down activities for about an hour.
- *Have a bedtime ritual.* This will help cue your mind to begin thinking 'sleep'. For example: lock up, have a hot bath, get some supper, brush your teeth, change into your nightclothes, set your timer or alarm clock, turn off the lights.

When you are in bed

- *Use your bed only for sex and sleep.* Avoid reading, watching television or working in bed. (For a minority, such habits are not a problem, so experiment.)
- *Relax your body and mind.* The *breathing-focus* technique (p. 126) is a good way to relax both. Choose to postpone problems; if you worry you might forget them, reassure yourself by writing them down.
- *If you wake during the night,* let yourself fall asleep again. If you are still awake after fifteen minutes, get up (see pp. 138–9 for suggestions on what to do next).

When you get up in the morning

What you tell yourself immediately on rising can have a major impact on how you feel during the day. If you tell yourself you hardly slept a wink so you're going to feel lousy all day, you are likely to create a self-fulfilling prophecy.

On the other hand, suppose you think: 'Well, I haven't slept as well as I would have liked, but I have got some rest. If I give myself a push and get moving now, I will most probably perk up and get through the day OK', this self-fulfilling prophecy will do you a lot more good.

Dealing with particular sleep problems

Even when you have rectified any problems of basic sleep hygiene, you may still find you have trouble sleeping. Scan the subheadings that follow to identify any difficulties relevant to you, then read about what you can do to improve matters.

Trouble falling asleep

- During the day, don't nap (unless experimentation tells you otherwise) or take stimulants.
- Two to four hours before going to bed, have a meal high in complex carbohydrates — cakes, jam, ice cream, fruit pie, dates, figs, breakfast cereal, bread, milk, chocolate, potatoes, spaghetti, etc.
- Don't go to bed until you are ready for sleep — tired, relaxed and calm.
- If you feel tense in bed, use a relaxation strategy. The *breathing-focus* technique (p. 126) is particularly effective.
- When in bed, say to yourself: 'I'm tired and ready to go to sleep.' When you experience disconnected thoughts or muscle twitching, think: 'I'm falling asleep.'
- If you are still awake after about fifteen minutes, get up and follow the suggestions in the next section (*Lying awake in bed*).
- Finally, don't sleep late in the morning, including at weekends.

Lying awake in bed

If you have had trouble sleeping for some time, your mind will have come to associate being in bed with being awake. You need to break this unhelpful association.

- *If you find yourself staying awake at any time during the night for more than about fifteen minutes,* don't lie in bed any longer. *Get up.* Go into another room. Stay up for as long as you feel necessary, probably about twenty to thirty minutes. When you feel tired, go back to bed. Here are some things to do while you are up:

– Read something boring.
– Have some herb tea, a milky drink, a bread and honey sandwich or some milk and cereal.
– Do something physically tiring: ironing, cleaning, sorting out.
– Do crossword puzzles, logic exercises, anything that requires the brain to work in short, sharp bursts. (But don't read an exciting book that will leave you wondering what happens next.)

• *Repeat this process* as often as you need to during the night, and for as many nights as it takes for the wakefulness habit to be broken.

Restless sleep

• Experiment with avoiding sleep during the day.
• Exercise vigorously (preferably before 4.00 p.m.).
• Identify and deal with any underlying anger.
• Establish a good pre-bedtime routine.
• Immediately before bed eat a high-carbohydrate snack.
• Get up one hour earlier than usual.

You wake early in the morning and cannot get back to sleep

• Are you sleeping during the day, going to bed too early, having a strong drink during the evening or taking sleeping tablets?
• Check out the possibility of depression (p. 26).
• Cut out any daytime or early-evening sleeping.
• Establish a good pre-bedtime routine.
• Don't go to bed until you are absolutely ready for sleep. Make yourself stay awake until then (though not with stimulants such as caffeine or nicotine).
• Abstain from alcohol, stimulants and sedatives while establishing your new sleep pattern.

Trouble getting up in the morning

Identify and deal with the cause:

• *Your sleep is disturbed during the night.* Identify and rectify the cause(s).

- *Your room is too dark in the mornings.* Allow for some morning light to enter (while keeping your room reasonably dark at night).
- *Heavy caffeine use.* Keep your intake down, using the guidelines already outlined (p. 134).
- *Use of sleeping pills for an extended period.* Sleep medication suppresses a key phase of sleep essential to refreshing the bodily system. Refrain from taking pills, or see the guidelines later in this chapter (p. 143).
- *Consumption of alcohol close to bedtime.* This has a similar effect to using sleeping pills. See earlier guidelines (p. 134).
- *Irregular sleep routine.* Your internal 'body clock' is confused. Regularise your routine.
- *Stress* — emotional or physical. Use the relevant strategies in this book to deal with it.

Sleep times out of sync with the rest of the world

Going to bed late and sleeping late is usually a habit people get into over a period of time. To break it, you need to reverse the process, step by step.

- *Set your alarm fifteen minutes earlier* on the first day. That evening, go to bed fifteen minutes earlier. Every few days, bring your alarm and your bedtime further forward until your hours are back to normal.
- *Do the reverse of this.* Progressively *delay* your bedtime and getting up time until you eventually work your way round the clock. This will obviously require some reorganisation of your lifestyle, but it works better for some people.

Once you have reset your internal clock, keep to a regular routine.

Noise

- *Reduce the noise if possible.* Install double glazing, negotiate with neighbours about parties or the use of stereos, call the noise control officer if all else fails.
- *Isolate yourself from the noise.* Insert earplugs, or try a 'white noise generator' (an electronic device that blankets other noises in the room).
- *Use psychological coping strategies.* If you change what you tell yourself about noise, you will tolerate it better. Identify especially any anger which keeps you awake. It is possible to sleep despite high levels of noise (children and young people are often not bothered by it).

- *Distract yourself from the noise.* The *breathing-focus* relaxation technique (p. 126) can help you do this. There is also a strategy I call *absorbing*. I dislike noise, and have tended in the past to get angry, regarding it as something that 'shouldn't be there'. Unfortunately, demanding that the noise not be there simply fixated my attention on it! Now I allow myself to be aware of the noise, then visualise myself 'absorbing' rather than rejecting it. This makes the paradox work in the opposite direction: by accepting noise, I find it less bothersome.

Teeth-grinding

- *Get a dental check.* Often some repairs are all that is needed.
- *Try this simple technique.* Clench your teeth firmly for about five seconds, then relax for five. Repeat five or six times a day. Continue for about three weeks, or until the grinding stops. If the problem persists, consult your doctor for further advice.

Your bed partner

- *Snoring.* A person usually snores when they sleep on their back. Try moving them so they are on their side. Raise the head of the bed, or have them sleep with several pillows. Put an object like a golf ball in a sock and sew it to the back of their nightclothes. Encourage them to seek medical advice.
- *Teeth-grinding.* See the suggestions above.
- *Leg-jerking.* Consult a doctor.

Worrying

- *Worrying keeps you awake.* Schedule a 'worry time', when you deliberately focus on your worries. Try to make this about the same time each day. If you worry that you might forget to worry, reassure yourself by writing a list of the things you are bothered about.
- *You remember worrying matters in the night.* Keep a pen and paper by your bedside. Firmly remind yourself that the middle of the night, when you are not fully awake, is the wrong time to try and solve problems. Make a note of what is bothering you and commit yourself to dealing with it the next day.

Jet lag

If you travel, say, from Auckland to New York, at 11.00 p.m. local time your body 'thinks' it is really 3.00 p.m. and not yet time for sleep. Dealing with jet lag warrants a book of its own, but here are a few tips:

- Avoid alcohol during the flight.
- Drink plenty of non-alcoholic fluids to minimise dehydration.
- If possible, arrange to arrive at your destination late in the day, and switch immediately to the new time.
- Organise a light schedule for your first few days in the new time zone.

Shiftwork

Shiftworkers are highly likely to experience sleep problems. There are a few measures you can take to lessen the ill-effects:

- Try to eat meals at the same time each day.
- Get four or five hours' sleep at the same time each day, no matter when this is.
- Avoid using stimulants to stay awake.
- If possible, keep to the same routine even on the days you are not working.

Unpleasant dreams

Probably everyone has bad dreams from time to time. It is possible, though, to increase their frequency and scariness by telling yourself they are awful, intolerable and must not happen.

- *Carry out a Rational Self-Analysis* (p. 80) on your thoughts about the dreams. Accept the dreams as a discomfort you can tolerate, rather than something you can't stand. If you see them for what they are — just dreams — they will most likely start to reduce in frequency.
- *If this doesn't work*, it may be wise to see your doctor to check for the possibility of a medical condition.
- *Beware of using sleeping pills* as a quick and easy solution. They may suppress the dreaming phase of sleep, but when you come off them there could be a rebound effect, with a resurgence of dream sleep dominated by bad dreams.

Use of sleeping pills

The use of sleeping pills is a controversial subject. Sleep medication is helpful for some people under some circumstances, but the consensus at the present time is that it is usually appropriate only for short-term use.

The main problem with such medication is that the sleep it brings is unnatural. The dreaming phase is suppressed, and if this goes on for long, you will suffer during the day. There is also the danger of addiction, with consequent withdrawal stress. Moreover, some sleep problems can actually be made worse by sleep medication.

If you plan to use sleep medication, you would be wise to see a doctor rather than simply purchase an over-the-counter drug.

Overcoming the blocks to managing your sleep

Do what works for you

This chapter contains many potentially useful ideas. Treat them as suggestions, not directions. What works for other people, even the majority, may not work for you. It is important that you apply the principle of *self-knowledge* (p. 54):

- Experiment to find what suits you. For example, try napping during the day, then try staying awake, and see which helps you sleep best at night.

Motivating yourself

Persevering with the strategies presented in this chapter may test your motivation. You could, for example, find yourself lying in bed awake because it would be 'too uncomfortable' to get up and break the pattern. You will probably find it stretches your discomfort tolerance to keep getting up during the night. It will become even harder if you find that a few nights of doing this doesn't fix the problem. The key principles here are *tolerance for frustration and discomfort* (p. 60), *long-range enjoyment* (p. 62) and *emotional and behavioural responsibility* (p. 66):

- Remind yourself that getting up is simply uncomfortable, not awful or unbearable, and that facing up to the discomfort is in your interests. This will help you persevere until you have broken the pattern of lying in bed awake.
- Resist the temptation to sleep in on weekends and holidays by noting

that the short-term pleasure this gives you will disrupt your long-term sleep routine.

- When you feel tempted to use the quick fix of sleeping pills, remind yourself that getting to sleep straightaway may come at the cost of longer-term sleep problems.
- Finally, don't blame other people or circumstances for your sleep problem: put yourself in control of solving it.

Don't let anger keep you awake

Sometimes there will be elements in your environment that make it hard to sleep, such as noise from neighbours, or an adolescent who stays out at nights. Apply the principle of *acceptance of reality* (p. 75):

- If you can do something to change the situation, do it.
- If you cannot, you have two options. You can rail against your circumstances, tell yourself 'this shouldn't be happening', and stay angry and awake. Or you can accept you dislike the situation and would prefer it to be otherwise, but acknowledge there is no Law of the Universe that says it 'should not' be as it is.

When you stop upsetting yourself over reality, you will significantly increase your chance of getting a good night's sleep in spite of it.

Attitudes to sleep by

Self-defeating beliefs	*Rational alternatives*
I must be able to feel and function at my best every day, so I need a good night's sleep.	Demanding I be at my best every day will only make me uptight. Then I'll be less likely to perform at my best — and less able to get to sleep!
There's little I can do to handle the tiredness, irritability, anxiety and poor functioning that results from poor sleep.	There's a lot I can do to deal with the consequences of not sleeping well — if I take responsibility for finding solutions and putting them into practice.
It's awful to have a sleepless night, and I can't stand the way I feel the next day.	It's uncomfortable — not a source of 'horror'! I dislike the way I feel after a poor sleep, but I can (and do) stand it.

I must get a good sleep every night.	I'm more likely to get to sleep if I stop demanding I do.
I should be able to sleep well every night, no matter what.	It would be great to sleep well every night no matter what — but I'm a human being, not a robot that can be switched on and off!
Insomnia is ruining my ability to enjoy life and stopping me from achieving my goals.	Insomnia harms my wellbeing, but it will only ruin my life if I let it.

Further reading on sleep

Nicol, Rosemary. *Sleep Like a Dream: The Drug-Free Way.* Sheldon Press, London, 1988.

Tyrer, Peter. *How to Sleep Better.* Sheldon Press, London, 1978.

13
Maintain a Support System

Getting support from other people can play a significant role in reducing the effects of stress.[1] Talking problems over seems to ease emotional tension. It helps unload annoyances before they become major issues. Putting concerns into words often clarifies them, even if the person one is talking to says little or nothing. A second opinion often contributes to a clearer understanding of a problem. And it just seems to make a difference to know one is not alone in facing life's adversities.

Where to get support

Support may come from a range of people, including your partner, close friends, acquaintances, relatives and coworkers. What kind of people will you find supportive? Probably people you can trust, who are good listeners, and who respect your competence but can be honest with you when necessary.

Where to look for support

There are many places to make contact with potential supporters. Some common ones are:

- at work
- social clubs
- church groups
- special interest clubs and societies
- adult education classes
- local neighbourhood support groups
- specialised support groups

The four levels of relating to other people

Support operates at more than one level. It is useful to see friendship as falling into four main categories:

146

1. *Acquaintances* — people you know casually. You may have many of these.
2. *Friends*, varying in closeness, of which you will have a smaller number.
3. *Close friends* — usually one or two, rarely more.
4. *Intimate relationships*, e.g. with a lifetime partner. (If you have more than one of these, you may be adding to your stress!)

Different levels of self-disclosure are appropriate for different relationship levels.

1. At the most superficial level, we disclose little about ourselves — probably only basic facts: what we do, where we are from, the things we enjoy, or some current activity.
2. At the second level, we go beyond presenting information to stating opinions and sharing our own beliefs, attitudes, values, concerns and judgements, thus exposing more of ourselves.
3. At the third level, we communicate our emotions, hopes, dreams, loves, joys and sorrows, which are more personal to us than our opinions. We tend to communicate at this level only with people we trust.
4. At the fourth and highest level, we communicate not only our opinions and emotions, but also our inner secrets. Usually, we reserve this level for our very closest relationships.

Sometimes people are afraid to make new contacts because of anxiety about how much they think they have to reveal of themselves. But you are not obliged to tell everyone everything about yourself. Nor do you have to tell any particular person very much; it is for you to decide what you reveal once you have got to know someone and decided how close you want to become. Ultimately you do not have to expose yourself totally to anyone — not even your lifetime partner.

Contrary to what some counsellors, self-help books or devotees of encounter groups will tell you, you won't become mentally ill if you keep some things to yourself. In fact, you might do better to suppress specific tendencies — such as an inclination to be sarcastic, for instance — when you are around other people, while you work at replacing them with more constructive ways of communicating.

An introduction to social communication

Is conversation a problem for you? What follows are some practical suggestions for getting to know other people.

Starting conversations: questioning and listening

Start by making simple observations and asking 'routine' questions that are easy to answer.

- Notice something positive about the *other person*, mention it and ask a question:
    - Draw attention to something they are wearing and ask where they got it.
    - Mention something they are doing and ask how or where they learned to do it.
    - Comment on something they are carrying — a musical instrument, for instance, or an item of sports equipment — and ask about it.
- Comment on, or ask something about, the *situation or place* in which you find yourselves:
    - What does the other person think of the gym, dance hall or conference venue?
    - Do they live or work nearby?
    - Try to be positive in what you say about the situation.
- Only use closed questions ('Are…?' 'Do…?' 'Who…?' 'Where…?' 'Which…?') to break the ice. Move quickly to open-ended questions ('How…?' 'Why…?' 'In what way…?'). These help keep the conversation moving forward.
- Listen out for information the other person volunteers and use it as a basis for follow-up questions.

Above all else, listen actively. Don't worry about how you are coming across — concentrate on what the other person is saying. Relate what you say to what you hear from them.

Keeping the conversation going: getting more information

Keep listening actively:

- Concentrate and use inviting body language — eye contact, smiling and nodding.

- Listen out for facts, opinions, feelings or other information the person gives you that you can use to keep the discussion going.
- Use words and phrases that encourage the other person to keep talking: 'What happened then?', 'How did you react to that?', 'What led you to that conclusion?', etc. Summarise every now and again: 'You mean that…', 'What you're saying is…', etc.

People communicate in many ways — with the words they use, through their clothing, body language, personal behaviour and activities. Keep your eyes and ears open for useful information you can use to keep the conversation going.

Deepening the conversation: self-disclosure and further questions
When the time is right, disclose something about yourself:

- Share personal interests, big events in your life, rewarding experiences, your work, interesting aspects of your background.
- When appropriate, move on to sharing your hopes and goals.

Remember, as we have seen, that there are different levels of self-disclosure. You do not have to tell everything about yourself. Don't overload someone you have just met. Be open, but regulate what you disclose. And be realistic about yourself. Don't exaggerate your good qualities or hide your faults. Sharing your goals and struggles is what will bring you closer to others.

Continue getting to know more about the other person:

- What interests them?
- What do they get enthusiastic about? Explore areas such as work, hobbies, career goals, trips, sports, social causes.
- As before, look for messages you can read from jewellery, clothing or whatever they might be carrying.

As you find out more about the other, offer more about yourself. Relationships develop and deepen as people share of themselves in a more or less equal fashion.

General principles for effective communication

- Take every reasonable opportunity to practise these skills — talk with fellow-travellers, checkout operators, people in queues and so on.
- Be active rather than passive. Don't wait for other people to say hello — greet them first.
- Make your body language friendly — smile, lean forward, make eye contact.
- Don't worry too much about what *you* are going to say. Instead, concentrate on what *the other person* is saying. The trick to being a good communicator can be summed up quite simply: learn to *listen*.
- Some rejection is inevitable, but there are things you can do to minimise it. Watch for the right time to approach someone. Look for any signs that they may be prepared to receive contact from you. Be friendly and direct, rather than hesitant. And keep in mind that when you do happen to be rejected, it isn't catastrophic. Accept the situation gracefully. Don't dwell on it, just move on.
- Present yourself positively. Most people do not want to relate to someone who comes across as whining or negative. A smile or a compliment will cost you nothing, but will usually pay dividends. This does not mean you should be insincere, or flatter to deceive. In the long run, it is not wise to present yourself as something you are not. What it does mean is making the effort to offer others something about which they will feel good. They will then be more likely to feel like offering something in return.
- Pay people compliments on such matters as their clothes, sports ability or musicianship. Practise by complimenting at least one person every day.
- When someone compliments you, never play it down — accept the compliment.

Making a start on building support

Get active

Support systems will not usually come to you: you need to get moving and seek them out. Start by listing your hobbies, preferred leisure activities, other areas of personal interest and work activities. Then develop a list of possible ways to make contact with new sources of support.

To structure this exercise, use a form like this:

Hobbies, leisure activities, interests	Possible contacts
Photography	Jim across road in camera club

Work activities	Possible sources of support
Employee performance review	Michael in Human Resources Dept

Right now, develop one specific assignment for approaching a potential source of support. Each week, go through your list and approach another contact. List new contacts as you think of them.

Keep in mind that this process requires active looking. It may take a while; only some of the many people you meet may be suitable. But the longer you work at it, the more you will increase your opportunities.

Overcoming the blocks to using support

Do you accept yourself?

Rating yourself negatively will show in self-defeating behaviours like avoiding closeness, seeing yourself as undesirable and acting accordingly, or failing to look after your body and mind. You can help yourself with the principle of *self-acceptance and confidence* (p. 55), coupled with some *Rational Effectiveness* techniques (Chapter 8):

- If you worry that others may reject you or let you down, remind yourself that you would still be the same person — *you* would not change. Acknowledge any shortcomings in your social skills, but rate your *behaviour*, not your *self*.
- Use the positive attributes you have to attract new friends and sources of support, and recognise that what you have to offer is of some value. Your confidence will increase as you work at making improvements so that you have more to offer others.
- Put these new ways of viewing yourself into practice with *shame-attacking* (p. 88) and *acting out of character* (p. 89). Confront any fear of revealing yourself to others by doing it (sensibly, of course). Ease your anxiety with *Rational Self-Analysis* (p. 80) and *imagery* (p. 86).

151

Overcome social anxiety

Are you overly self-conscious in social situations, preoccupied with your own appearance and behaviour? You probably fear being rejected or looking foolish or embarrassing yourself. Underlying these fears will, usually, be self-defeating beliefs such as: 'I must perform well and be seen as a competent socialiser', or 'I couldn't stand doing anything that might lead to embarrassment.' *Tolerance for discomfort* (p. 60) is the key principle here:

- Remind yourself that while you won't like rejection or embarrassment, it will not kill you.
- Confront your social anxiety with *exposure* (p. 88). Deliberately get into social situations. Stay with the situation and the resulting discomfort. When you ride out your discomfort, you will discover that you can bear it after all.
- Try *distracting* yourself from your self-consciousness by actively *listening* (p. 148) to the person with whom you are communicating. (As well as reducing your anxiety, this will help you get started with building relationships.)
- Apply *relaxation* techniques (p. 119) to any physical tension.
- Prepare yourself in advance for social situations. Use *imagery* (p. 86): imagine yourself in the situation you fear, disputing your irrational anxiety-creating beliefs and using effective communication skills. *Role-play* (p. 90) new ways of communicating with someone who will give you feedback on how you are doing.

Face any fears about getting close to people

Do you tend to avoid more than superficial involvement with others? You may fear rejection, have trouble trusting people, or fear getting hurt if you become too close. Awfulising and discomfort intolerance are most probably involved. You see rejection as 'awful', to have a confidence revealed as 'catastrophic', or to begin a relationship and then lose it as 'unbearable'. Three of the rational principles will help you here — *tolerance for frustration and discomfort* (p. 60), *risk-taking* (p. 64) *and acceptance of reality* (p. 75):

- View rejection and embarrassment as unpleasant or undesirable, rather than 'awful' or 'unbearable'. They won't kill you. You can stand it when others do not reciprocate or behave badly.
- Relating to others is always a risky business, and you will be rejected

or let down from time to time. But remind yourself that the risk is worth the potential gains, and is a much better option than the certainty of getting no support at all by playing it safe and not reaching out.

- When friends and acquaintances turn out to be less than perfect, and let you down and say or do hurtful things, accept that they are just like you — fallible human beings. Then you will be able to go on relating to them.

Is jealousy a problem?

Do you get upset when friends and acquaintances spend time with other people? Jealousy is usually based on lack of self-acceptance. You demand that your friends always put you first, so you can be constantly reassured that, because you are the most important person to them, you must be OK. This creates anxiety, and places restrictions on others they are unlikely to tolerate for long. The key principles here are *self-acceptance* (p. 55), *self-direction and commitment* (p. 68) and *emotional responsibility* (p. 66):

- If you accept yourself, you will have little need to feel jealous about others.
- Work on directing your life in all areas. Then you will be less likely to become dependent on a particular relationship.
- Remember that your emotions are caused not by what your friends do, but by what you tell yourself about their actions.
- Involve yourself in absorbing activities that don't involve the people toward whom you feel jealous.
- Confront any jealousy with *exposure* (p. 88). Actively encourage those of whom you are jealous to pursue social contacts and interests other than yourself.

Overcoming loneliness

Fear of being alone often leads to overconformity or destructive relationships. Also, if you cannot enjoy your own company, it is unlikely others will. Loneliness compounds itself.

Loneliness actually has little to do with being alone. It is possible to feel lonely in a crowd. Loneliness results from self-defeating beliefs about being on one's own — in particular, beliefs about one's own 'unworthiness'. The key principles here are *self-acceptance* (p. 55) and *commitment* (p. 68):

- Accepting yourself will reduce any need to have other people around you to 'make you feel good'.
- Develop hobbies and interests that do not depend on other people but which you find absorbing.
- Confront loneliness with *exposure* (p. 88). Get used to your own company by deliberately arranging to be alone and filling your time with satisfying activities.

Dependency issues

If you lack confidence and self-acceptance, this may lead to dependent behaviour — constantly seeking reassurance, or demanding more of relationships than they can provide. At the other extreme, are you overly independent, an 'I don't need anyone' individual? Superindependent people may appear strong on the outside, but often they have an underlying fear of getting close to others or of becoming dependent. Key principles here are *self-direction* (p. 68), *moderation* (p. 65) and *emotional responsibility* (p. 66):

- Make sure you are directing your own life in all respects; then, even though you actively seek the support of others, you can be confident you remain your own person.
- Set and maintain appropriate boundaries which even close friends do not cross. Allow people only so far when it comes to your time, body, money and property. Conversely, avoid overloading your supporters, by setting limits on the demands you make of them.
- Remember that you, ultimately, have control over your own emotions, so you can accept support from others confident that, whatever happens, you will still be able to cope with your feelings.

The importance of reciprocity

When two or more people relate, it is because each perceives the other has something to offer.

There are people who take but do not give. Do you hold absolutist expectations of friends and acquaintances? Do you, for example, expect them to be there seven days a week for support, company, baby-sitting or whatever else you may want of them? Do you think they should be prepared to lend you money or help in other ways without question? Do you demand they be willing, in the name of friendship, to take whatever you do or say to them without complaint, or to sacrifice their own desires and wishes in order to fulfil yours?

On the other hand, there are those who give but do not (apparently) take. I call this the 'social worker syndrome'. Are you available to help when your friends want you, but make out that you expect nothing in return? Your selfless behaviour may really be just the opposite. It puts you in a one-up position over others, allowing you to boost an otherwise poor ego. This is yet another sign that self-acceptance is lacking — you 'help' others to convince yourself you are OK. Unfortunately, your 'selflessness' adds to your stress, as the unequal nature of the relationship means you give support but don't receive it in return.

Enlightened self-interest (p. 58) is the key to avoiding both of these problems. Meaningful relationships are based on mutual self-interest, or reciprocity:

- Give — in order to receive. Attend to others' interests so they will be encouraged to attend to yours.
- Consider not just what others have to offer you, but what you have to offer them.
- If you want help without having to give anything in return, see a professional counsellor.
- If you want to be a social worker yourself, attend an accredited course of training, then build up a clientele separate from your social circle.

Show respect for others

Do you find it hard to respect others? If so, you will have trouble relating to them. Lack of respect for other people leads to inconsiderate behaviour and intolerance, but it usually reflects a lack of respect for oneself. Putting down other people is, most often, an attempt to boost a shaky ego. The principles that apply here are *self-acceptance* (p. 55), *emotional and behavioural responsibility* (p. 66) and *long-range enjoyment* (p. 62):

- If you accept yourself, you will find it easier to accept others.
- Don't blame others for your feelings or circumstances, then you will be less likely to alienate them. Take responsibility for dealing with the emotions that result from your own self-defeating thinking, rather than expecting others to do it for you.
- Be able to choose, when appropriate, to forgo immediate satisfaction of your desires in order to build better relationships that will provide support in the long term. Propositioning a colleague for sex, or taking out your anger on a friend, may seem like a way to ease your

frustration in the short term, but could lose you a source of support in the longer run.

Don't put on a front

Do you change how you talk and act according to whom you are with? The trouble with this is that no-one ever gets to know just who you are, and you may attract people with whom you are not compatible. *Self-knowledge* (p. 54) is the key principle:

- Know yourself.
- Don't try to be all things to all people.
- Let others get to know you as you really are (even though you may choose to improve aspects of yourself over time).

Support or isolation?

Self-defeating beliefs	*Rational alternatives*
It would be awful to share something of myself with others and have them turn it against me.	It would be disappointing but hardly cause for terror! Although I wouldn't like it, I would survive it.
I must be absolutely sure that other people are trustworthy before I can open myself up to them.	It is desirable that other people be trustworthy, and I will be sensible about who I trust, but demanding an absolute guarantee will ensure I never trust anyone.
I couldn't bear to let myself get close to someone and then have them reject me, so it isn't worth the risk.	If I don't take the risk, then I *guarantee* isolation and lack of support. Rejection is disappointing, but hardly unbearable. After all, it has happened in the past and I'm still alive!
True friends should be prepared to do things for you without expecting anything in return.	Why on earth would anyone want to relate to me (or anyone else) as a friend unless they also got something out of the relationship?

I couldn't stand the embarrassment if I made a fool of myself in front of other people.	While I dislike embarrassment, it doesn't kill me. Telling myself it's unbearable only makes it feel worse than it needs to.
It's unbearable to feel lonely, so I must have other people around me.	Feeling lonely is unpleasant, not 'unbearable'. And being alone is not what causes loneliness. I would do better to learn to be more comfortable with my own company.
True friends are either there for you totally or they're not worth having.	Where is it written that friends should be totally committed? I can enjoy what I get from people with all levels of commitment to me.

Further reading on maintaining a support system

Gabor, Don. *How to Start a Conversation and Make Friends.* Sheldon Press, London, 1983.
Hauck, Paul. *How to Love and be Loved.* Sheldon Press, London, 1983.

14
Act Assertively in Your Dealings with Others

You will be better able to maintain a support system, and in fact to use most of the strategies in this book, if you know how to get across to other people what you think and feel, what you want and what you don't want.

What is assertiveness?

Assertiveness is the process of communicating in such a way that you are heard clearly by others, while respecting what they think and feel. There are three main aspects to being assertive: (1) asking for what you want, (2) saying 'no' to what you don't want, and (3) expressing your thoughts and feelings.

Assertiveness, contrary to what many think, is not aggressiveness. You are being assertive when you ask directly and clearly for what you want. You are being aggressive when you demand that it be given or use threats. Assertiveness, while being direct, respects other people and takes their interests into account.

Assertiveness can be applied in many areas of life, such as:

- Declining inappropriate or inconvenient requests.
- Communicating concerns to others and asking for changes.
- Asking for what you want.
- Expressing appreciation.
- Negotiating.
- Stating your point of view.

Why be assertive?

Assertiveness is highly relevant to stress management. If you stand up for yourself, people are more likely to respect you and treat you accordingly. Being able to say no will help you avoid putting other people's priorities ahead of your own. Getting others to change how they act toward you will mean fewer stress triggers in your life.

By acting assertively, you can avoid the resentment that builds up through holding in feelings such as annoyance or irritation. Resentment often expresses itself in physical symptoms, and the build-up of emotions can eventually overflow in response to even a minor provocation. It is better (at an appropriate moment) to express feelings assertively at an early stage.

Communicating your concerns assertively will also help you avoid aggressiveness. Expressing what you feel or want in an inappropriate manner alienates others. Being assertive is more likely to win their cooperation.

The assertiveness questionnaire

The following questionnaire will help you identify any unassertive tendencies you may have. Give each statement a score, using the scale provided:

I do this most of the time	I do this fairly often	I do this half the time	I do this now and again	I hardly ever do this
5	4	3	2	1

Doormat behaviour
__ 1. I want something but fail to ask for it.
__ 2. I don't say anything when someone behaves in a way I dislike.
__ 3. I do something I don't wish to do, or which is highly inconvenient to me.
__ 4. I modify my speech and behaviour to conform with those around me.
__ 5. I ask permission of others before I do or say things.
__ 6. I apologise for things even when I'm not responsible.

Holding in emotions
__ 7. I tell myself it's wrong to feel angry towards another person.
__ 8. When I'm annoyed, I hold it in rather than express it.
__ 9. When someone is behaving towards me in a way I dislike, I get very tense in my body.
__ 10. I feel resentful because I believe I'm being forced to do something or deprived of what I want.

Aggressiveness
__11. I ignore the interests of others in what I do and say.
__12. I blame and accuse others when things go wrong.
__13. I threaten others to get them to cooperate with me.
__14. I feel hostile towards others and try to get back at them.

Calculate your scores for each section as follows:

Add your scores for questions 1 to 6 here: _____, then divide this total by 6: _____ (this is your *doormat behaviour* score).

Add your scores for questions 7 to 10 here: _____, then divide this total by 4: _____ (this is your *holding in emotions* score).

Add your scores for questions 11 to 14 here: _____, then divide this total by 4: _____ (this is your *aggressiveness* score).

A score of 3 suggests you may have a problem; 4 or 5 indicates that some work in the area concerned is a priority.

A primer on assertive behaviour

Now that you have identified any unassertive tendencies, the next step is to see what you can do about them. There are four key requirements for effective assertiveness:

1. You know the difference between passive, aggressive and assertive behaviour.
2. You have specific techniques to communicate assertively what you wish others to hear.
3. You accept and respect both yourself and others.
4. You are able to think rationally before acting.

What is assertive behaviour?

You are being *passive* when your response is to say nothing, or you are vague and unclear. You are being *aggressive* when you demand that others give what you want or attempt to force them to comply. You are being *assertive* when you communicate in a clear and direct fashion that shows respect for yourself and the other people involved.

The chart that follows gives some examples to illustrate the three types of behaviour:

Passive	*Assertive*	*Aggressive*
You say yes to something you don't want to do.	You say no, express your regret, and say you hope they'll find another solution.	You tell them to get lost and stop being a pain in the neck.

Passive	Assertive	Aggressive
When someone asks you out, you say you aren't available that particular evening.	You gently tell the person you're flattered but don't feel the same way, so it wouldn't be helpful to go out together.	You tell the person they're pathetic and you'd never go out with anyone like them.
When seeking information, you give up when told it's inconvenient.	You politely explain why you believe you're entitled to the information, and keep repeating your request.	You abuse or threaten the other person.
You say nothing when an employee has done a particularly good job on a project.	You tell the employee he's done a good job and express your appreciation.	You tell the employee that you expect him to keep it up and do even better next time.
You let your flatmate smoke in the house even though you've made a no-smoking agreement.	You remind your flatmate of the agreement, but agree to a compromise whereby she smokes on the patio outside.	You tell your flatmate she's an unthinking bitch and has twenty-four hours to get out.
An employee is regularly late for work, but you say nothing in case you upset him.	You explain privately that you want him to be at work on time, or to let you know if he's delayed.	You tell him, in front of other staff, that if he's late once more he'll be dismissed.
You'd like to ask out a coworker, but you just hint that such-and-such a restaurant is a good place to eat.	You approach your coworker, say you've heard about a great restaurant, and ask if she would like to go there with you.	You say that as you've helped out with her work she should return the favour by going out with you.

Passive	**Assertive**	**Aggressive**
You'd like to express your view in a discussion, but fear the others will consider it stupid.	At an appropriate juncture in the discussion, you say what you think.	You interrupt and tell the others their views are stupid and that yours is the only correct one.
You feel hurt about something but pretend it doesn't matter.	You say: 'I feel hurt about what you did, and would like to discuss it with you.'	You say: 'You hurt me, and you're a bastard.'

Expressing concerns

- Deal with issues as they arise. Don't let your feelings build up.
- Take responsibility for your own feelings and what you want changed. Use 'I' statements: 'I feel hurt' and 'I'd like you to...', rather than 'You hurt me' or 'You should...'
- Comment on a person's *behaviour,* not their total being. Criticise only what can be changed.
- Be specific. Tell others exactly what they are doing about which you are unhappy. Be explicit about what you would like them to do instead.
- Don't minimise your concerns by being apologetic or down-playing their seriousness, but avoid overgeneralising: 'You *always*...', 'We *never*...', 'It's *totally*...', etc. are almost invariably exaggerations.
- Take care with timing. Raise a contentious issue only when other people are not upset or preoccupied. Resist the temptation to launch straight in; set the scene to get a more constructive result.

Asking for what you want

To get a positive response, make requests simply, clearly and directly, so others are clear about what you want. Here are some examples:

- 'I'd like more information about this medication, please.'
- 'What I'd like most from you is a listening ear.'
- 'I'd really like to go out with you.'
- 'Please let me know when you're going to be late.'

Sometimes you will have good reason to persist. On other occasions it will be appropriate to take no for an answer. Learn to discriminate.

Assertive people are reasonable in what they ask for and how they put it across. They sensibly evaluate when it is in their interests to persist or to desist. And they know that a willingness to compromise will often get them more of what they want in the long run.

Saying no to what you don't want

If you are unsure about someone's request, ask them for further information or an explanation. Don't say yes until you are sure you are satisfied. When there is pressure on you to give an answer, say you will get back to them. If they cannot wait, you may be better just to say no.

When turning someone down, be succinct, decisive and clear with your refusal, so the other person is in no doubt as to where you stand. But be polite, too; then you will be more likely to get your message across without ill-feeling. Here are some examples:

- 'Thanks for offering me a special deal on the deluxe model, but I'll stick to the basic machine I specified.'
- 'I'm flattered that you want to go out with me again, but I don't think we're suited to each other, so I'll decline. But thank you anyway.'
- 'Thank you for asking me to join your committee, but it doesn't fit my plans. However, I wish you well in your endeavours.'
- 'I like working in a place where we all feel good about each other, but please don't hug me when we're alone in the office.'

You can choose to explain your reason for saying no, but you don't have to. Sometimes an explanation is appropriate, sometimes it isn't required. On some occasions it may actually be best not to give one — for example, when you suspect the other person is likely to argue with you.

If necessary, keep repeating your position in a reasonable but firm manner until the other person gives up. Keep in mind that if you resist for a while, then give in, they will keep at you even longer next time.

Handling criticism

The first thing to do when criticised is *stop*. Restrain yourself from doing what comes naturally, which for most people is to get defensive. Instead, question your critic. Ask for more information. Get them to be specific about their concerns. When you are satisfied you understand what they are unhappy about, ask them to be clear about what they want instead.

Acknowledge that you have heard your critic, and show that you understand their concern (even if you disagree with it). Then explain how you see things. Don't counterattack with another criticism, or condemn the other person, if you think they are mistaken.

What if your critic is overdoing it? Tell them how you feel when they overgeneralise about your actions or rate you as a person. Explain how you would like them to speak to you when they have concerns.

What if the criticism is warranted? Wear it gracefully. Being able to take criticism and acknowledge shortcomings is a sign of maturity. People will respect you for that.

General principles concerning assertive strategies

- Pick your time. Requests will get a better response when the other person is relaxed rather than pressured or preoccupied. Sometimes it may be wise to arrange a meeting in advance so that both parties can be prepared.
- Be specific when describing a problem and the solution you envisage.
- Take responsibility for what you want and don't want. Say 'I'm concerned about...' or 'I'd like you to...', rather than 'You mustn't...' or 'You should...'. Use 'I' language rather than appeal to 'universal laws' that everyone 'should' know about.
- Start with the lowest appropriate level of assertiveness, then work up to higher levels if necessary. For example:
  - 'Thank you for asking, but I don't think it would work for us to go out together.'
  - 'Thank you, but no.'
  - 'I've already said that I won't be going out with you. Please don't ask again.'
- As the preceding example shows, you will sometimes need to be persistent. In fact, there is a technique called the *broken record*, which is commonly taught on assertiveness-training programmes. Make sure, though, that you do not carry persistence to the point of becoming aggressive.
- Be prepared to listen to others. People are more likely to cooperate when they feel they have been heard. Sometimes, too, you may learn something that will lead you to change your position.
- Show others how it would be in their interests to cooperate with you. Point out the advantages of what you are trying to achieve. People are

more likely to change when they see it will be to their advantage, rather than because someone thinks they 'should'.

- It may be necessary to explain why it would be against someone's interests not to cooperate. You might, for example, point out to an adolescent that if they fail to get home by dinner time, their meal will be thrown out. But use such negative reinforcement only when the positive hasn't worked. And never make a threat unless you are prepared to carry it out, otherwise you will be training people to take no notice of what you say.
- Finally, be prepared to compromise. You will get more of what you want when you are prepared to meet other people halfway.

A programme to increase your assertiveness

For assertiveness to do you any good, ultimately you need to 'walk the talk'. Here's how you can go about putting the head-learning into practice.

Role-playing

You will find assertive behaviour easier if you practise before using it in the real world. *Role-playing* (p. 90) is a good way to do this. All you need is a trusted friend or colleague who will play the part of another person. Describe the person to your helper and coach them in how to react. Keep repeating the role-play until you feel you have got your approach right.

Exposure

When learning how to be assertive, don't just wait for opportunities to arise — set up practice ones. Then you can prepare for them and have more control over what happens while you are learning. (See also p. 88.)

1. Start by making a list of things you could do. Here are some examples:
   - *Express your feelings or views.* Write about an issue to your local newspaper. Each day, tell someone about an interesting thing you are doing. Ask someone to explain a view they have expressed. Speak up about something you dislike. Protest about something you disagree with. Put forward an idea.
   - *Ask for what you want.* Ask someone to help with a task. Request something from a person in authority. Ask a question. Ask for service. Ask for feedback on something you have done. Invite someone to go out with you. Start a conversation with a stranger on a

bus or train. Arrange with your family that they do their own thing while you do something by yourself.

- *Say no to what you don't want.* Decline a request you see as inconvenient or unreasonable. End a phone conversation when you feel like it. Talk to someone whose behaviour you dislike. Confront someone who tries to make you feel guilty. Withdraw from a commitment you have made but do not want. Terminate a boring conversation.

2. Grade the items on your list according to how much anxiety you feel about each one.
3. Action at least one item from your list each day:
   - Start with the items that cause you the least anxiety, gradually moving up the list to higher-anxiety situations.
   - Prepare yourself beforehand by using *Rational Self-Analysis* (p. 80) or *imagery* (p. 86) to deal with any dysfunctional thoughts and emotions that might hinder you.
   - Reward yourself for each item you confront.
   - When you do slip up and act passively or aggressively, don't rate yourself. Instead, analyse your lapse to identify the cause and see how you can avoid repeating the mistake in future.

Overcoming the blocks to practising assertiveness

Many people learn assertiveness strategies but never put them into practice or quickly give them up. The reason is simple. They have learned how to *act* assertively, but they have not identified and changed the self-defeating *beliefs* that stopped them being assertive in the first place. They may also have picked up some new irrational beliefs while they were learning to act assertively! Let's see how these blocks can be overcome using key rational principles and *Rational Effectiveness* techniques (Chapter 8).

Be aware of your values and goals

If you don't know what you want out of life, or are unclear about your values, you will have trouble deciding how to react when people want your time, money or body. *Self-knowledge* (p. 54) is a key principle if assertiveness is going to work for *you*:

- Have *goals* (see Chapter 9). Know what you want out of life, in both the short and long term. Then you will make better decisions about when to say yes or no and how far to go in pursuing your wants.

Combat self-downing

If you believe you are not as good as other people, or worry about their opinion of you, you will hold back from saying what you think or asking for what you want. *Self-acceptance and confidence* (p. 55) is the key principle here:

- Understand that you do not need to be any particular kind of person to justify being assertive.
- Remember that even when others react badly to you when you attempt to be assertive, or you realise you have handled a situation wrongly, you are still the same person as you were before.
- As you learn and practise assertive skills, be confident that no matter what the result, you have the ability to cope with your emotions when things don't work out.
- Use the technique of *paradoxical behaviour* (p. 89). Deliberately give yourself one treat each day for a while to disprove the idea that you must be 'deserving' to have or do pleasant things. As far as possible, make these treats requests you ask of other people.

Raise your tolerance

Do you think you 'should' or 'must' always have things the way you want? Low frustration tolerance will create unnecessary conflict with others. Low discomfort tolerance may cause you to view the risks involved in behaving assertively as too much to bear. The principles that will help you are *risk-taking* (p. 64) and *tolerance for frustration and discomfort* (p. 60):

- Remember that nothing in life is guaranteed. Asserting yourself will not always produce the results you would like, but to get any results, you need to take the risk of an occasional bad reaction.
- Note that while risk is uncomfortable and you (naturally) don't like it, it is not awful or intolerable. You can, and do, stand it.
- Increase your frustration tolerance by challenging any demands that other people or the world be as you want them to be. Be prepared to ask for what you want, but without demanding that you 'must' have it.
- Use *exposure* (p. 88) to increase your tolerance. For a while, carry out one new assertive action a day. Prepare yourself with *imagery* (p. 86), *role-playing* (p. 90) or a *benefits calculation* (p. 86).

Make sure your self-interest is balanced

Total self-centredness will ultimately put you offside with those around you. Total other-centredness will keep you living for others and denying yourself. Either way, you will end up with less of what you want. *Enlightened self-interest* (p. 58) will help you get things in balance:

- If you acknowledge you are a self-interested human being, and view that as normal and acceptable, you will be more likely to seek what you want and decline what you don't.
- Keep in mind that it is in your interests to take into account the interests of others. This will help you seek to build an environment in which people meet each other halfway and everyone gets something of what they want.

Let others take responsibility for their own feelings

Do you think you cause other peoples' emotions? Guilt will stop you acting assertively through fear of 'hurting' their feelings. Help yourself with *objective thinking* (p. 72), *emotional and behavioural responsibility* (p. 66) and *self-direction* (p. 68):

- Rid yourself of the magical belief that you somehow have power over other people and can miraculously cause them to feel emotions. Remember that other people create their own emotions in the same way you create yours — through what they tell themselves.
- As well as letting others be responsible for their emotions, take responsibility for your own. Avoid blaming anyone for the way things are. Instead, get on with the job of changing what can be changed.
- Set your own goals and act in ways that help you achieve them, rather than live according to the goals of others. (Take care, too, that you are not choosing a particular lifestyle simply to show opposition to authority figures, such as your parents.)

Keep your assertiveness in proportion

Do you believe you 'must' act decisively each and every time your 'rights' are infringed? This could be keeping you constantly alert for any perceived encroachment, and lead you to compulsively assert your rights even when it would be better to let something go. *Long-range enjoyment* (p. 62), *moderation* (p. 65) and *flexibility* (p. 71) are key principles here:

- Resist the temptation to gain short-term relief by using aggressive-ness to get what you want. Forgoing immediate satisfaction will often help you get a better deal from other people in the long run.
- Don't become obsessed with being assertive. Avoid carrying it to the point where you are always on the lookout for situations where your 'rights' are being infringed and where you 'must' get your own way, no matter what the cost.
- Treat each situation as different. Think before you respond, rather than always saying either yes or no. Keep in mind, too, that assertive-ness is not a cure for every problem, but is simply one means of improving the quality of your existence.

The problem with 'rights'

Paradoxically, one of the common blocks to behaving assertively is brought about by many assertiveness-training books and programmes themselves. In the 1960s and 1970s, the idea was promoted that there are a number of basic 'rights' upon which people are entitled to insist. The theory was that if people could be encouraged to believe they had these rights, they would feel more justified in acting assertively. These rights now have an almost religious status.

As Harold Robb has observed, however, there are some practical prob-lems with the notion of rights.[1] People who believe they are absolutely entitled to what they want can become dogmatic. They can feel victimised when deprived. A number of people all standing on their rights can create unresolvable conflict. *Assertive paralysis* occurs when a belief in one's rights conflicts with the knowledge that nowhere are these rights guaranteed. Worst of all, pushing the notion of rights means less emphasis on teaching people other, more valid, reasons for acting assertively.

What is the solution? It is simple. *You don't need a 'right' to be assertive!* If you want to change your mind, you can — simply because you decide to. If you don't want something, you can say no — simply because you don't want it. You can ask for what you do want simply because you want it. You don't have to fret about whether you have a right to it.

There is a much more effective way to evaluate your wants. Instead of considering your rights, evaluate *what is in your interests*. Ask yourself: 'Is it in my interests, in the long as well as short term, to...(change my mind/say no/ask for this)?'; 'Will it help me achieve my goals?'; 'Will it contrib-ute to both my immediate and my longer-term happiness?'

This is not the same as unbridled self-centredness — that would be just as bad as the rights approach. Sometimes you will decide it is in your longer-term interests to agree to do something you would rather not, or to refrain from asking for something you would like. Principles such as *enlightened self-interest* (p. 58) and *long-range enjoyment* (p. 62) will provide you with more useful guidelines than the dubious and problematic notion of 'rights'.

Self-defeating v assertive thinking

Unassertive beliefs	*Self-directed beliefs*
Other people are more important than me.	Where is it written that some people are more important than others?
To be assertive is to risk discomfort, so I'd better play it safe.	If I don't assert myself, I guarantee bad results for my life in general.
You should never do anything that might make another person feel bad.	It's thoughtful to consider other people's feelings; but, ultimately, human beings cause their own emotions.
You should always give other people a good reason for what you think, do or say.	While it may sometimes be appropriate to do so, nowhere is it written that people always have to justify what they do.
I must always be consistent, decisive and constant, so that others can depend on me.	I can change my mind — simply by choosing to. It would be sensible, though, to consider how this might affect others.
I should always try to help someone who has a problem.	I can choose to help, but I don't have to find solutions to other people's problems.
You should avoid being a burden to others by asking for what you want or sharing your problems with them.	It's good for people to help each other when help is offered out of choice. Other people are just as able as I am to say no if they don't wish to grant my request.
People should always act in a correct fashion, and it's embarrassing and shameful to make mistakes or blunders.	It's human to make mistakes. I can take responsibility for mine and still accept myself; and I can accept others when they get things wrong.

Unassertive beliefs	*Self-directed beliefs*
People should always treat me with fairness and justice.	I like the world to be fair and just, but where is it written I should be exempt from reality?
I must never reveal my stupidity by asking questions or failing to give an answer.	It's OK, and often helpful, to say 'I don't know', 'I don't understand' or 'I'd like to think about it.'
Other people must always think well of me, and it would be unbearable if they didn't.	I'd prefer other people to like me, but I can stand it — and act assertively — when they don't.
I can get people to like and respect me if I ignore what I want and just do things to please them.	If I act like a doormat, I'll be treated as one. People usually have more respect for those who know what they want and can say no to what they don't.
You can't turn people down when they want something from you.	It's for me to decide what I do with what's mine. I don't have to give my property, body, time or energy when I don't wish to, or feel guilty about saying no.
It's selfish to put your own wants before those of others.	Notions of 'selfishness' or 'unselfishness' just lead to guilt and manipulation. Enlightened self-interest is a far better idea, not just for me, but for everyone.

Further reading on assertiveness

Dyer, Wayne W. *Pulling Your Own Strings.* Avon Books, New York, 1978.

Ellis, Albert, and Lange, Arthur. *How to Keep People from Pushing Your Buttons.* Citadel Press, New York, 1994.

Faber, Adele, and Mazlish, Elaine. *How to Talk so Kids Will Listen and Listen so Kids Will Talk.* Avon, New York, 1982.

Hauck, Paul. *How to Do What You Want to Do.* Sheldon Press, London, 1976.

Hauck, Paul. *How to Be Your Own Best Friend.* Sheldon Press, London, 1988.

Hauck, Paul. *How to Stand Up for Yourself.* Sheldon Press, London, 1981.

Jakubowski, P., and Lange, A.J. *The Assertive Option: Your Rights and Responsibilities.* Research Press, Champaign, IL, 1978.

Manthei, Marjorie. *Positively Me: A Guide to Assertive Behaviour.* Methuen New Zealand, Auckland, 1981.

Smith, Manuel J. *When I Say No I Feel Guilty.* Bantam Books, New York, 1975.

15
Keep Stimulation and Variety in Your Life

The human body requires constant change in order to function. Consider your sense of smell. When you scent a rose, you are struck by the lovely perfume. After a while, though, the intensity diminishes as you become used to it. If you go to a different type of rose, you can smell with renewed acuteness, because your nose finds the sensation fresh and novel.

The mind works on the same principle. It constantly needs restimulating. You will probably have noticed how reading a book is at first absorbing, but then your concentration begins to dull. When you put the book down, however, and do something else for a while, you come back to it fresh.

Lack of variety and stimulation leads to boredom. This state of mental weariness and discontent is itself stressful. Boredom may lead to depression, or to high levels of frustration.

A degree of challenge and stimulation is important for good mental health, but when stress rises too high, performance begins to decline. We need challenge — and the occasional break from challenge.

How you can create stimulation and variety

Introduce variety into your workday

'Work' is what you do to earn a living or maintain yourself and your dependents. It may involve housework, a business you operate from home or a job in an office or factory.

Introducing variety into your workday in the form of *pauses* — breaks at regular intervals through the day — can improve your concentration and functioning. The extent to which you can do this will depend on how much control you have over your time and responsibilities.

If you have little control, try and get away from your work area whenever you have a scheduled break. Do something entirely different. Have a brief nap, take a short walk, get some refreshments, read a book, write a letter, socialise with a colleague, listen to music, use a relaxation technique.

Time-out every few hours will refresh you, keep you alert and help you maintain peak efficiency.

If you have greater freedom to plan your day, use it to alternate tasks that take time. 'A change is as good as a rest' may be rather shop-worn but still holds true. Take regular breaks to talk to colleagues, get a drink of water or even just walk to the filing room to get away from your desk.

If you are a homemaker, plan your day so you are not constantly doing the same thing. Take regular breaks from routine tasks like cleaning and cooking, or home maintenance activities like house-painting or redecorating (unless you find them absorbing).

Have interests outside of work

Have some pursuits that regularly take your mind in a different direction from work. This will help you return to your labour refreshed and with increased efficiency.

Common pursuits include:

- sport (be it organising, playing, coaching or supporting)
- an absorbing hobby
- do-it-yourself projects
- organising events (e.g. a family reunion, concert, dance, play or sporting fixture)
- researching (a topic of interest, family history, etc.)
- expanding your areas of interest and aptitude (e.g. learning a musical instrument, attending wine-tasting classes, meeting new people)
- an absorbing commitment (e.g. volunteer work, committee membership, political activity, writing a book)

Other pastimes, for relaxation and simple enjoyment rather than more enduring purposes, include:

- outdoor activities (walks, beach visits, picnics, etc.)
- reading, going to the movies, visiting places of interest
- socialising with family or friends
- treats (a long bath, a massage or facial, getting out the photo album)

Take planned holidays

If you wait until you 'have the time', holidays may never happen. If you don't plan ahead, you may waste precious time. Don't wait for holidays to happen — organise them.

Holidays don't have to be spent away from home. You could plan an interesting do-it-yourself project, arrange picnics or visits to a museum or art gallery, call on friends you don't normally get to see, or pursue any number of special activities.

Sometimes you might want to get away from it all. Planning is especially important when bookings need to be made or arrangements set in place to care for your house, pets or children. Going away can range from a world trip to an inexpensive camping holiday.

Whatever you do, the trick to taking time off is planning. Don't just drift along. Organise your time off work and plan what you are going to do. Then do it.

Finding new things to do

From time to time, vary your pursuits and try out new ones, including some you haven't previously thought of. There are many places you could look for ideas.

Your local Public Relations Office may have a list of events taking place over the next year. Keep an eye on notice boards in supermarkets, church halls, museums and other public places. Many organisations advertise in public libraries.

Seek out local community groups which organise activities ranging from craftwork, sports and eating-out in small groups, to voluntary help with such matters as budget advice or telephone counselling. Free local newspapers are often a rich source of advertisements for these groups.

If you have lived in the same place for some time, you may have come to take it for granted and could be surprised to discover just what is happening all around you.

Getting into action

If you are not used to taking time-out, it may be especially important to plan recreation rather than wait until you 'have time'. Planning ahead can help you combat the tendency of most human beings toward inertia, which we will discuss shortly.

Recreation activities sheet

An activity planner like the one on the next page will help you get started. Plan some kind of recreational activity for the next four weeks and record what you intend to do each day in the relevant box. Some days you will have time for only a short activity, on other days you will be able to set aside time for a longer one. It is fine to repeat an activity, as long as it does not become so repetitive it grows boring.

Monday	Tuesday	Wednesday	Thursday	Friday	Saturday	Sunday
Go for a walk	Play with the kids	Read a novel	Go for a walk	Watch a movie	Have a picnic	Go for a drive

At the end of each week, review what you have done. Tick the activities you carried out, put a cross by the ones you missed. Analyse why you missed these. There may be a valid reason — for example, an unexpected opportunity to pursue a better alternative. But watch out for invalid reasons, like 'didn't have time' or 'didn't feel like it' (especially any that appear more than once). Plan how you can get round any blocks.

Keep using the plan-chart until you find you are routinely making time for recreation.

Overcoming the blocks to an enjoyable life

Given that human beings are usually motivated to seek pleasure and avoid pain, it may seem strange that we should need to consider blocks to self-enjoyment. The reality is that many people have self-defeating attitudes and behaviours that get in the way.

Don't let guilt stop you

If you feel guilty about pleasure, you will keep putting work before enjoyment or other people ahead of yourself. Beliefs such as the following will often underlie guilt: 'It's wrong to put pleasure before work', 'You can't relax till all the work is up to date', 'You should always put others first', or 'I don't deserve to enjoy myself.' Key principles to apply here are *self-acceptance* (p. 55), *self-direction* (p. 68) and *enlightened self-interest* (p. 58):

- Get rid of the idea that you have to 'deserve' pleasure or 'earn' it.
- Seek activities for enjoyment's sake rather than for boosting your ego.
- Watch out for any overcompetitiveness, fear of failure or anxiety about your reputation that creeps into your recreational pursuits.

- If you accept yourself, you will be able to feel comfortable with your own company and thus enjoy a greater range of recreational options.
- For variety and stimulation to do you much good, they need to be the kind you want, not what suits someone else. There are times, of course, when compromise is called for; for example, a parent who has just worked a six-day week and not seen much of his or her family is probably well advised to go with them on a picnic even though surfing the Internet has more appeal. But make sure you are not constantly fitting in with others' plans to the exclusion of your own.

Make the time

Most of us, if we are going to find time for anything, need to *make* that time. If you wait until you 'have time' for recreation, it will hardly ever happen. Are you constantly responding to external demands rather than taking control of your time?

Some people get caught in the 'spontaneity trap'. They believe it is only possible to enjoy themselves when recreation happens unintentionally. To plan enjoyment seems to be artificial. Consequently, they rarely break out of the grind of work and responsibility. Key principles that will help here are *self-knowledge* (p. 54), *self-direction* (p. 68) and *acceptance of reality* (p. 75):

- Know what you like and know what you want to get out of life. Then you will put your time and energy into activities that will bring you the most rewards.
- Don't wait until you have time — *make* time to do the things you really enjoy. How you spend your time is a matter of how you choose to set your priorities. What you think you 'have' to do is, in reality, a choice. You can choose to make enjoyable activities a high priority. See Chapter 16 if you need some help with managing time.
- Accept that you cannot do everything. If you are like me, your work will never be up to date (whatever that means!). Accepting this reality will help you get on with putting more variety and stimulation into your life.

Confront lack of confidence and fear of failure

Do you distrust your intelligence or abilities? If so, you will restrict the range of activities open to you. A strong fear of failing will make you less likely to try new things. Or it could lead you to become overcompetitive, which will take much of the enjoyment and relaxation out of your recreation. When we say we are afraid of failing, what we really mean is that we fear disapproval from others and our own self-downing. Sitting underneath this is lack of self-acceptance. Key principles here are *self-acceptance and confidence* (p. 55) and *risk-taking* (p. 64):

- Remember that you don't become a different person when others disapprove of you, and that failing does not make you 'a failure'.
- Know what you are capable of and what your limits are. Then you will make sensible choices on recreational activities without unnecessarily restricting your options. Do you have a disability? Changing attitudes towards disability, and advances in equipment such as lighter and stronger wheelchairs and prostheses, are opening up a widening range of activities and leading to an increase in confidence among people with disabilities. Maximise your options, but don't set yourself up for disillusionment with unreasonable expectations.
- There are risks involved in stepping out and trying new things. But you guarantee lower satisfaction if you play it safe and only ever pursue what you already know. Risk-taking is part of a stimulating and varied life. Don't just think about doing something different — try it out. Some things will work for you, some will not; but there is no way of knowing which will or won't without trying them.

Be able to be alone

If you have an excessive fear of loneliness, you may cut yourself off from many enjoyable activities that involve being alone. Spending time with other people is important to most human beings; but spending some time alone will provide variety and refreshment in your life (making your socialising, when you engage in it, even more enjoyable). See page 153 for suggestions on overcoming loneliness.

Avoid compulsiveness

If you take up an enjoyable activity and become obsessed with it, then it will lose its pleasure and become a new source of stress. Do you exercise compulsively, spend all night on the Internet or find you cannot put down a book or magazine until you have read it right through? Help yourself with the principles of *moderation* (p. 65) and *flexibility* (p. 71):

- Exercise is good for you — in moderation. Enjoy watching television — but don't become a couch potato. Take inspiration from involvement in a political or community action group — but remain able to see other points of view.
- Don't get in a rut. Avoid doing things the same old way all the time. Go to work by a different route some days. Skip the cafeteria now and again; bring your lunch from home and eat it under the trees. Go camping in a different place next holidays. Be able to move from one activity to another in order to maintain your freshness, enjoyment and efficiency.

Break out of inertia

It is often easier to think about doing something than to do it, even when the activity is potentially enjoyable. Human beings seem to have a natural tendency towards inertia. Underlying this, mostly, is low tolerance. Four principles will help you in this respect — *tolerance for frustration and discomfort* (p. 60), *long-range enjoyment* (p. 62), *commitment* (p. 68) and *emotional and behavioural responsibility* (p. 66):

- Remind yourself that while overcoming inertia might be uncomfortable, it won't be fatal — and it will get easier the more you do it.
- Acknowledge the reality that highly satisfying pursuits, such as learning a musical instrument, writing a book or building a house, take time to develop and bear fruit — but will increase your long-term enjoyment of life.
- People benefit from pursuing a variety of activities. With some, like watching a movie, you will have only a superficial commitment. But greater satisfaction will come from absorbing yourself in one or a few undertakings on a long-term basis.
- Blaming your boss or partner because you don't seem to have time for yourself is a sure way to remain stuck. Take responsibility for your own action or lack of it. When you see that the power to make your life more interesting is in your own hands, you will have taken the first step toward doing something about it.

Boredom or stimulation?

Self-defeating beliefs	*Rational alternatives*
It is self-indulgent and weak to seek pleasure when there is work to be done.	Variety and stimulation are important to physical and mental health, and they help me work smarter rather than harder.
I must always get my work up to date before I play.	Sometimes it is appropriate to discipline myself to complete a task before playing. But my work can never be 'up to date'. And taking breaks makes me more efficient in the long run.
It is easier to go along with whatever happens rather than try to change anything.	It is only easier in the short term. Inertia leads to boredom and depression. Facing the immediate discomfort of getting moving will make life better in the long term.
I can't take time for myself because other people make it impossible.	Other people may make it difficult, but ultimately I choose whether I fit in with them or seek what I want.
I don't have the time to take time-out.	How I allocate my time is, ultimately, a matter of personal choice.

Further reading on stimulation and variety

Ingham, Christine. *Life Without Work: A time for change, growth and personal transformation.* HarperCollins Publishers, London, 1994.
Roberts, Paul. 'Risk'. *Psychology Today*, 27:6 (Nov–Dec), 50–84, 1994.

16
Manage Time to Achieve Your Goals

By now you will have realised that many of the strategies for managing stress — exercise, relaxation, recreation, etc. — require time. Managing time effectively, therefore, is a key stress-management strategy. Unfortunately, it is one that many people study but few practise. One reason for this is a misunderstanding as to what time management is about.

Many people think it is a dry subject concerned solely with efficiency, but this is not the case. Time management is not just about efficiency — it is about *effectiveness*. It is about managing time *in order to achieve one's goals*. It is about planning and prioritising so that your time gets spent on *what is really important to you*.

Will time management make any difference to your life?

Know why you want to manage your time

When deciding how to use your time, there are three questions to ask yourself regularly:

1. Where do I want to go in my life?
2. What is the best way to get there?
3. Am I doing that?

If managing your time is to serve any useful purpose, you need to know what you are working toward. That means being clear about your values and overall goals, and your monthly, weekly and daily objectives. A goal-oriented approach will keep you in touch with some basic principles of time management:

1. What is important and what is urgent are not necessarily the same.
2. The idea is to achieve your goals by working smarter, not harder.

180

3. People who achieve their goals don't 'find' time for what is important — they *make* time.
4. Effective time management is enlightened; that is, you take into account the aims and goals of other people, knowing this is the best way to achieve your own.

Do you need to improve your management of time?

Complete the following time-management test. Score 0 for 'never', 1 for 'sometimes', 2 for 'often':

___ I think I have used my time poorly.
___ I seem to be working under constant pressure.
___ It seems there are not enough hours in the day.
___ I feel overloaded.
___ I feel frustrated because I am not able to finish the jobs I regard as important.
___ I find myself doing things I don't want to do.
___ I spend evenings and weekends working to meet deadlines.
___ I miss deadlines.
___ I find it hard to trust subordinates with tasks, so I do them myself.
___ I have trouble making decisions about what to do.
___ I tend to lack time for personal relationships, rest and recreation.

Add up your scores. If your total is 0–7, you are probably managing your time reasonably well. A score of 8–15 suggests some work on time management would be useful. If you scored 16 or more you would be wise to make this area a priority. Note the items on which you scored higher so you can give them particular attention.

The practice of effective time management

Know what matters

The key to time management is to spend your time on what is important. What is important is what helps you achieve your goals.

Take the advice of time-management consultant Alan Lakein and continually ask yourself 'Lakein's question': 'What is the best use of my time right now?'[1]

This question applies to all areas of your life — recreation, family, work. Worrying about something you forgot to do at the office is a poor use of time when you are relaxing with a book. Thinking about your next project is a poor use of time when your partner is trying to communicate about a family problem.

Keep in mind that there are four categories of time usage:

1. Important and urgent.
2. Important but not urgent.
3. Urgent but not important.
4. Not important and not urgent.

People often miss the point that what is urgent is not necessarily important. The idea is to concentrate your efforts on categories (1) and (2).

Be aware, too, of the 80/20 rule: '80 percent of the benefit comes from 20 percent of the time and effort expended on a task. The other 20 percent of gain takes 80 percent of the effort and time.'[2] Put your time where it counts. Don't strive for perfection when 80 per cent accomplishment will do the trick. Five 80 per cent tasks add up to 400: one 100 per cent task adds up to only 100.

Plan

Planning is one of the keys to managing time rather than it managing you. Plan for the next year, month and week, then for each day. List tasks that are aimed at achieving your objectives and put them in order of priority.

- *Ignore things that are of low usefulness* in achieving your goals. Emphasise what you want to accomplish (the outcomes) rather than what you do (the inputs).
- *Plan all significant projects* (including home and social events). List all the things that need to be done and their deadlines. Set a starting time for each. Estimate how much time you need, and add one-third to cover any unexpected problems. If appropriate, transfer specific items to your diary. If you have a planner-type diary, keep your project lists in it.
- *Break down goals and larger tasks into manageable steps.* This will help you get started, and you can see how you are doing as you cross off each completed item.
- *Prioritise tasks in terms of their importance.* Remember that important tasks are those that move you towards your predefined goals and objectives.

Planning principles

- Be flexible in your planning; allow extra time for unexpected interruptions.
- Make sure your plans are realistic.
- Don't schedule more into a day than you can reasonably expect to do.
- Allow adequate time for travelling where this is necessary, so you are not driving fast in a panic, or getting stressed in a queue at a ticket counter.
- Keep a notebook and pencil with you, in your pocket or handbag. You can then write down any items you want to recall later on.
- Keep a diary and record in it all your appointments or items to remember (both personal and work related). Look at the diary every morning.

How to get started

- If you have broken down large tasks into a number of smaller, manageable steps, it will be much easier to get started than if you are confronted with a few huge and overwhelming projects.
- Carry out the tasks on your daily list, starting with the top-priority ones, then moving to those further down. Cross off each item as you go — the sense of completion will be motivating.

How to get finished

- *Work efficiently.* Have a proper filing system at home as well as at work. Every year, throw away unneeded papers, put any you wish to keep in a separate box, and leave in your filing system only those with which you are currently working or which you may need to consult.
- *Keep your desk or work area uncluttered.* Do you prefer to keep out of sight work that is waiting to be done? If so, list 'to do' items in your diary or planner, then file the relevant folders and papers where you can find them when it is time to work on them. Alternatively, if you are a 'visual' person who prefers to keep everything in view, organise your 'piles' into categories and colour-coded folders.
- *Set deadlines on specific subtasks.* This will help you avoid any perfec-

tionist tendency to waste time getting a task 'just right'. One proviso, though: don't make finishing an absolute demand. Sometimes you may benefit from setting a task aside, doing something else, and coming back to it later when you are refreshed.

Creating extra time

You can achieve your objectives faster by creating extra time. Here are some tips (highlight the ones you plan to follow):

- *Free yourself from time-wasters.*
  - Low-importance tasks, e.g. unnecessary paperwork or reading, jobs that don't contribute to the fulfilment of your objectives.
  - Looking for items you cannot find due to a poor filing system or hoarded clutter.
  - Inadequate equipment, e.g. slow computers, inefficient software, having to share equipment that is much in demand.
  - Unnecessary travel or waiting; duplication of effort; unnecessary or poorly run meetings.
  - Inadequate information, e.g. task requirements unclear, people not available for discussion.
  - Leaving tasks unfinished then having to redo them from the beginning.
  - Reduced speed, e.g. through dreaming, fatigue or poor concentration.
  - Low-priority interruptions, e.g. casual telephone calls, people dropping in, distractions of a nice view or noisy environment, extended coffee breaks, idle conversation. Be prepared to tell people you are busy. Put a sign on your door when you are unavailable.
- *Spend less time on tasks.*
  - Give yourself deadlines and stick to them.
  - Be aware of dawdling signals, such as daydreaming, reading the same words twice, talking to other people, and so on.
  - Handle paperwork once: read it, decide if any action is required, then do it or file it.
  - Make lists rather than leave files lying around.
  - Whenever possible, finish tasks at one sitting. This will be easier when you have broken down goals and large tasks into 'bite-sized' pieces.

- Ask yourself *Lakein's question* (p.181) regularly to check whether you are making the best use of your time.
- *Rid yourself of some tasks.*
  - Say no to requests and tasks that don't contribute to specific, desired objectives.
  - Delegate when you can.
  - Quickly scan rather than read your mail. Throw out or redirect items of low or no priority for you.
  - Keep minimal records; don't file items you can refer to elsewhere, unless they have special importance to you.
  - Simply wipe low-value tasks off the bottom of your 'to do' list.
- *Save time by spending money.*
  - Buy computer software that helps you work efficiently, even if it costs more than the package that came with your machine.
  - A fax machine may save time otherwise spent trying to catch people on the phone.
  - Would it be cost-effective to pay an outworker to take on some of your jobs, or a contractor to do your chores (such as mow your lawns), while you get on with tasks only you can do?
- *Do two things at the same time.*[3]
  - Listen to an inspirational tape while driving.
  - Plan an activity while doing the housework.
  - Use waiting time productively, e.g. read a file while waiting for someone to come to the telephone, take some reading with you to appointments in case you are early or your meeting is delayed, keep a list of quick tasks you can do whenever you have to wait.
  - But be careful not to overdo this, e.g. don't try to plan a project while playing with your children, or have so many things on the go you get distracted from finishing any particular one.
- *Spend less time on some activities.*
  - Forgo that lie-in and get up earlier in the morning.
  - Watch less television; plan your watching in advance and watch only high-priority programmes.
  - Shorten time spent socialising on the phone.

Making effective decisions

You can make better and quicker decisions by keeping in mind a few simple principles:

1. There is rarely a choice between a totally 'right' and totally 'wrong' decision. When evaluating options, consider which are preferable rather than which are 'right'.
2. It is usually better to risk making a faulty decision than to make no decision at all.
3. Sometimes it is appropriate not to decide at all. Be sure, though, that this is a deliberate choice and not simply avoidance.

A *benefits calculation* (p. 86) may be useful for breaking through decision-making blocks.

Managing yourself

Ensure you look after yourself, so you are capable of using your time effectively. Exercise, a healthy diet and time-out will all improve your ability to concentrate and think clearly.

During the day, stay alert by drinking water and having regular breaks in which you get up and move around, do stretching exercises, take short naps or use relaxation techniques.

Do you work best in the morning, afternoon or evening? Reserve your biological 'prime time' for your most important tasks or those that require good cognitive functioning.

Avoid inefficient or unhealthy practices. Don't routinely take work home or go to the office at weekends, or make overtime a habit. If you know you can continue with a task after hours, you will probably slow down during your normal working day.

A programme for moving to better time management

Identify your current problems

A useful first step toward improving your management of time is to find out where the time is currently going. Keep a daily time-use log for about a week, or at least a few days. Record the following items:

- Each activity.
- The time at which you began it.
- A rating of each activity's priority (in terms of how it contributes to your goals and objectives): 5, no importance; 4, low importance; 3, moderate importance; 2, high importance; 1, top importance.

- A rating of each activity's urgency: 5, needn't be done by any particular time; 4, get around to doing; 3, do sometime soon; 2, do as soon as possible; 1, requires immediate attention.
- If it is prearranged (put a tick), an interruption (put a cross) or something you initiated but without planning (put an asterisk).

You may find it useful to view your day as consisting of three parts: (1) from waking up in the morning to lunch time, (2) from lunch time to your evening meal, (3) from your evening meal to going to sleep. Fill in your log at the end of each segment. Here is an example:

Time	Activity	Importance	Urgency	Prearranged etc.	Comments
8.30	Checked voice mail	3	2	*	
8.35	Talked to Judith	5	5	✗	Enjoyed the chat, but too long
9.00	Team meeting	2	1	✓	Useful for communication
10.00	Jack re technical problem	4	1	✗	Could we avoid these emergencies?
10.25	Started production report	1	3	✓	Better to have started this earlier

At the end of each period, analyse your entries:

- *Did you plan your activities each day*, i.e. were your objectives clear, the tasks listed, and priorities set for each task?
- *Did the most important items receive the most attention?* What percentage of activities were important, urgent, both or neither? Did urgent items crowd out important items? Did you give the appropriate amount of time to each item? Which activities deserved more time than they got?
- *What could you have done more efficiently*, i.e. faster, in a simpler fashion, with less attention to detail?
- *What could you have avoided doing* by delegating, leaving until later or not doing at all?

- *What* time-wasters (p. 184) *could you eliminate or minimise?* Keep a list of your typical time-wasters. At the end of the log-keeping period, decide which are the most problematic and start work on them.
- *To what extent have you achieved your goals*, both your objectives for the day and your end goals? What goals appear to be neglected in your daily/weekly activities? To what extent are you putting your time into the goals that are important to you? What activities can you develop to move toward your goals more effectively?

Develop an action plan

- List the problems you have identified.
- Check their causes.
- Develop a solution for each one.

Start putting the solutions into practice immediately, and see how they work out.

Overcoming the blocks to using time-management strategies

Time management is, unfortunately, one of those skills that many people study yet fail to use. Here are some of the more common reasons. See which are true for you.

Stop procrastination

People put off difficult or unpleasant tasks for three main reasons: (1) *low discomfort tolerance* — they object to doing something which involves nuisance, unpleasantness or pain, so find the short-term relief of avoidance very attractive; (2) *perfectionism* — the job has to be done perfectly or not at all (in this case not at all); and (3) *low frustration tolerance* — they object to being told what to do, or believe they cannot do anything unless they 'feel' like it (an increasing problem in our feelings-focused world). The principle of *tolerance for frustration and discomfort* (p. 60) and some *Rational Effectiveness* techniques (Chapter 8) will help you get moving:

- Accept that discomfort and frustration are normal, inevitable and tolerable, then you will feel more like facing the tasks you see as unpleasant and discover that once you get started they are not so bad.

- Do a *Rational Self-Analysis* (p. 80) to uncover and change any self-defeating beliefs that get in the way.
- Do a *benefits calculation* (p. 86) on the short-term gain of avoidance versus the long-term gain of getting started.
- Use the technique of *paradoxical behaviour* (p. 89) — deliberately seek out unpleasant or worrying tasks to give yourself practice in facing them.

Stick with priorities

Do 'shoulds' and 'musts' distract you from your own priorities? Perhaps you believe that you should put the goals of other people ahead of your own. Or you may have a 'should' about hard work or duty which leads you to think that as long as you are keeping busy, everything is all right — irrespective of how much you are achieving. A variation on this is the fallacy that the harder you work, the more you get done.

- Note that working *smarter* rather than harder usually gets more done.
- Use *Rational Self-Analysis* (p. 80) to uncover and combat any demanding that distracts you from your priorities or keeps you working just for the sake of work.
- Complete the *time-use log* (p. 186) to see which of your activities are not achieving much.
- Use *paradoxical behaviour* (p. 89) to challenge the belief that you cannot do anything unless you 'feel' like it. Commit yourself to do one thing deliberately each day that you don't feel like doing. Keep this up for about a month, or until you think you have got the message.

Be able to say no

Fear of disapproval from others may be making it hard for you to set limits on how much they use you and your time. And if you believe that putting your priorities first would make you a bad or selfish person, fear of guilt will be bolstering your passivity. The key principle here is *self-acceptance* (p. 55):

- Remind yourself that *your* goals and time are just as important as anyone else's.
- Use *Rational Self-Analysis* (p. 80) to analyse any fears of disapproval or guilt.
- Practise *exposure* (p. 88) — commit yourself to saying no (or doing

other things you fear might lead to disapproval) at least once a day for a month.

- See Chapter 14 for more help on saying no.

Get the clutter out of your life

When you throw something out, you can never be certain it will not be needed sometime in the future. If your discomfort tolerance is such that you cannot bring yourself to get rid of papers or other items you are un-likely to need again, you may find yourself with such a collection of clutter that a lot of your time is spent simply sorting through it trying to find the things you want. Use the principle of *risk-taking* (p. 64) to break free:

- Don't get tied up in knots with protective measures like overdocu-mentation or unnecessary filing.
- Practise *paradoxical behaviour* (p. 89) — prepare and commit your-self to a plan to get rid of clutter within a set period. Action that plan on a daily or weekly basis, throwing out a bit at a time.
- Use *Rational Self-Analysis* (p. 80) to prepare yourself emotionally to throw stuff out.

Minimise distractions

Low discomfort tolerance may encourage you to daydream, or be distracted by things that catch your eye or attention, in order to put off difficult tasks. Apply the principles of *long-range enjoyment* (p. 62) and *moderation* (p. 65):

- Enjoy yourself in the present and take regular time-out. But resist the temptation to overindulge in passing pleasures — to watch just a few more minutes of television or to socialise instead of getting started on difficult tasks.
- Put distracting items like magazines, books or personal correspon-dence out of sight. Turn off the television and radio (unless you find background music a help).
- Keep *Lakein's question* (p. 181) in front of you where your eyes tend to alight when you slip into dream mode (I keep it on the top of my computer monitor).
- Retrain yourself with *punishments* (such as missing a favourite TV programme) when you have given in to temptation, and *rewards* when you go a full day keeping to your schedule.

Get things finished

Common reasons for not achieving closure on tasks include being diverted by other things, becoming too focused on the process of doing rather than on the desired outcome, and holding onto a task to wring the last bit of perfection out of it. *Moderation* (p. 65) and *risk-taking* (p. 64) will help you:

- Keep your goals realistic and settle for excellence rather than perfection. Remember the *80/20 rule* (p. 182). Go for what is good enough.
- Don't schedule more into the day than you can reasonably expect to complete.
- Handle a document once only — action it or file it.
- Break down large tasks into smaller bite-sized pieces so you can stay with one task until it is completed.
- If you have to leave a task unfinished, ensure you schedule a time to complete it later.
- Set deadlines and stick to them.
- Keep *Lakein's question* (p. 181) in front of you.

Be able to make decisions

There are four main reasons why you might have difficulty making decisions: (1) what you *want* to do conflicts with what you think you *should* do; (2) you engage in *black-and-white thinking* — seeking the 'perfect' solution or the 'right' decision; (3) *low discomfort tolerance* makes you avoid the risk involved in committing yourself to a decision; (4) *lack of self-acceptance* leads you to connect your 'self-worth' with making the 'right' decision. The key principles here are *risk-taking* (p. 64), *self-acceptance and confidence* (p. 55) and *flexibility* (p. 71):

- Set a time-limit on making decisions, with a commitment that if you have not decided when the time is up, you will toss a coin and go with whatever the coin shows. Before long you will want to make your own decisions rather than have the coin decide for you.
- Remember that making mistakes does not say anything about you as a *person*.
- Remind yourself that there is hardly ever a 'perfect' solution or only one 'right' course of action.
- Seek advice and opinions from others when you lack information, but ultimately trust your own judgement.

- Do a *benefits calculation* (p. 86) on the advantages and disadvantages of making a decision now or of continuing to put it off. Be honest about the real costs and risks of continuing to delay. You can also use this technique to make the decision itself.
- Use *Rational Self-Analysis* (p. 80) to uncover any internal demands that conflict with wants.

Deal with the demands of others

Your time may be filled solving problems for others, slavishly following workplace procedures or attending unnecessary meetings. This may be the result of fear of disapproval, distorted self-interest or lack of self-direction. Help yourself with the principles of *enlightened self-interest* (p. 58), *emotional and behavioural responsibility* (p. 66) and *self-direction and commitment* (p. 68):

- Remain focused on achieving your goals while bearing in mind that to be effective you need to take into account the goals and concerns of others. Keep the two in balance.
- Don't blame others because you fail to get everything of yours done. You will make more progress if you take responsibility for asserting yourself and seeking constructive changes in how your job or home life are managed.
- Don't leave it to others to organise your time and your life. Stay focused on your own goals and objectives.
- Make a strong commitment to stick with tasks and see them through, irrespective of what others are choosing to do with their time.
- Avoid solving problems for others unnecessarily; train people by your actions to think for themselves.
- Follow workplace procedures when you are required to, but don't let them enslave you. Often there is room for manoeuvre, allowing you to do your own thing as long as you 'pay the rent'.
- Don't devote more time than necessary to the personal goals of others, such as your supervisor or employer. Again, 'pay the rent', then act on your own aims and goals. Avoid unnecessary meetings arranged by others. Get people to be clear and specific about why they want a meeting, and be clear as to whether you need to be there. Consider sending a delegate in your place. Ask if issues that involve you can be discussed at a prearranged time so you can deal with them and go.[4]

Reduce fatigue

- Take regular breaks — go for a walk, use a relaxation technique, etc. Just do something different for a short while.
- Keep a glass of water handy and sip at intervals to keep refreshing yourself.
- To keep the blood circulating, regularly move your body during breaks and while sitting at your work station.

When time-management strategies don't seem to work

You may be trying to adopt strategies that don't suit your personal style. For example, some people benefit from having a clear desk, whereas others work best with all their files and materials out where they can see them. Are you slavishly trying to follow advice you got from a book, course or colleague, rather than experimenting with different ways of doing things and finding out what works for you? *Self-knowledge* (p. 54) and *flexibility* (p. 71) are the key principles here:

- To manage time *effectively* you need to know what you want to get out of life.
- To manage time *efficiently*, you need to develop strategies suited to your style. An excellent approach to time management that allows for individual differences is described by Sunny Schlenger and Roberta Roesch in their book *How to be Organized in Spite of Yourself*.[5]
- Be prepared to change direction if you realise you are pursuing the wrong objective or there is a better way to do something. If you accept that interruptions to plans and scheduling are a part of reality, you will be less upset by them.

Further reading on time management

Aslett, Don. *Clutter's Last Stand*. Writer's Digest Books, Cincinnati, Ohio, 1984.

Ellis, Albert, and Knaus, William J. *Overcoming Procrastination*. Signet, New York, 1977.

Lakein, Alan. *How to Get Control of Your Time and Your Life*. Signet, New York, 1973.

Schlenger, Sunny, and Roesch, Roberta. *How to be Organized in Spite of Yourself*. Signet, New York, 1989.

17
Manage Your Financial and Material Resources

Money does make a difference — up to a point. Having adequate money increases the range of options available for coping with stress. It can provide better access to sources of help, such as medical treatment, legal assistance and financial advice. How you use your money can affect the other dimensions of stress management — nutrition, social life, medical care, recreation and so on. Just having money available, even if it is not used, may provide a sense of security.

Many people, though, have plenty of money but still suffer from stress. And there are people with little money who manage stress very well. Clearly, then, money *by itself* is not the answer to stress management.

The crucial factor is one's attitude towards money. Your attitudes will influence both what you do with your money and how happy you are. Happiness is not determined by the money you have. It is determined by the beliefs you have about your money.

Values-based money management

Grady Cash, in his book *Conquer the Seven Deadly Money Mistakes*,[1] invites readers to answer the question: are you spending in harmony with your deeply felt values? Cash, a financial counsellor, has seen families spending significant sums of money in areas that they never mentioned in relation to their goals or dreams, and this expenditure was destroying their chances of realising their dreams. Over the years I supervised a community budgeting service, I observed the same pattern — people spending large amounts of money and, far from getting anywhere, often slipping deeper into debt and distress.

For your spending to be in line with your values, you need to know what those values are. You need to know what you want out of life. Otherwise your expenditure will be aimless, or just reactionary according to the pressures of the moment.

If you have not yet clarified your goals, see Chapter 9. Once you know what your goals are, base your spending decisions on them. Let's say you want to replace your old car. Do you buy a new car or a much cheaper second-hand one? If your most important goal is to achieve status, that might lean you towards the new car. But if your main goal is an overseas trip, you might choose the second-hand model. You can apply this principle of goal-based spending to all your expenditure — on housing, food, clothing, recreation and so on.

What do we use money for?

Grady Cash points out that money has no value in itself; it is useful only because it can be used to obtain four things:

1. *Material items.* These range from survival essentials, such as clothes, housing and food, to less essential items that may add to life, like a television set, a remodelled kitchen or a lovely garden.
2. *Services.* For example, electricity, medical treatment and car repairs, or being waited on at a restaurant or provided with entertainment such as a movie.
3. *Experiences.* Holidays, visiting new places, socialising, meeting new people, learning new things, etc.
4. *Feelings.* People want to have good feelings. Money cannot, of course, buy feelings directly, but, apart from purchasing the necessities of physical survival, people use money to obtain non-essential material items, services, and experiences primarily for the feelings that result from having these things. Is it possible that feeling good is, ultimately, what every human being is seeking?

Could you feel just as good as you do now, or even better, by adjusting the ways in which you use money? Which will give you the greatest happiness: spending on expensive restaurants, or eating out more cheaply and putting the savings toward sending a child to university? Upgrading to a more modern computer, or taking music lessons?

Using your money purposefully

Apart from essential spending to meet survival needs, what portion of your outgoings on material items, services and experiences is for the purpose of obtaining good feelings? Are your current spending patterns actually achieving that purpose, in both the short and long term? If you want to make the best use of your money, look at your expenditure in each of the four areas:

1. *Are you paying for material items you could get more cheaply or provide yourself?* Could you heat your house for less by investing in insulation? Could you grow your own vegetables or buy food in bulk and preserve it?
2. *Are you paying more for services than you need to?* Could you learn how to do household repairs or redecorating, get as much enjoyment from eating out at cheaper restaurants, or record television movies instead of hiring videos?
3. *Are you paying more for experiences than you need to?* Buying experiences is often a good use of money. An overseas trip, for example, is like an investment — you may benefit from the memories for many years. But if the point is to see one of the world's great cities, why not stay in a good bed and breakfast rather than an expensive hotel?
4. *Are there some things you could do to achieve greater happiness that involve spending little money*, or perhaps none at all? The ultimate goal is to feel good. Remember that your feelings are not simply the result of what happens in your life — they derive from *how you view* what happens.

The real secret to feeling good

If you believe you 'must' get what you want or 'must not' be deprived, you will be unhappy when you go without — and at risk of spending money you cannot afford. Let's say, for instance, you believe that you absolutely 'need' the love of your grandchildren. If they appear to be uninterested in you, you may try to buy their love with expensive presents.

Keep in mind that *money alone cannot buy you good feelings.* If the things on which you spend your money give you pleasure, and you can afford the expenditure, fine. But if you rely on money alone to feel happy, you are at risk, paradoxically, of achieving lower levels of happiness. This is because *to be happy, you need to work on what you think.* Relying on material items, services or experiences will divert your energy from what you really need to do — change how you view the events and circumstances of your life.

Does this open up ways in which you could use your finances more productively? Rather than spending money in an attempt to compensate for feelings of depression, would you do better to learn how to handle negative emotions? Could you stop trying to buy the love of other people and instead spend more time with them? Rather than squandering the rent money on a shopping spree to get back at a partner who treats you badly, could you learn instead how to be more assertive with them?

How you can achieve more with your resources

Prepare a budget

Many people misunderstand budgeting. They think it means simply cutting back on spending, but it is much more than that. Budgeting is, basically, *planning*. A budget is a financial plan in which income and expenditure are recorded and juggled until they balance.

Simply getting the figures to match, though, is not true budgeting. A budget is not just a means of balancing expenditure and income — it is a tool for helping in the achievement of goals. Whether the priority is to get out of debt or send a child to university, budgeting is something you can do all your life to maintain and improve the quality of your existence.

How do you prepare a budget? It is not as difficult as it may sound. Your first step is to make sure you are clear about your goals. Then you need to record your income and your outgoings.

Next, go through your outgoings. Do they reflect your important goals? Is there some allowance for emergencies and planned maintenance? Have you taken into account such matters as medical expenses? Is there any provision for your retirement? If any of these items are missing, put them in.

Now add up both your income and your outgoings. If you are fortunate enough to have more income than outgoings, you will be able to introduce some further spending on desired items, such as savings for a goal you thought you might have to postpone.

It is perhaps more likely, though, that your outgoings exceed your income. If so, you have several options. One is to increase your income. Think carefully here. Watch, for example, that you don't cater to a low-priority item, like paying off an expensive lounge suite, by taking a second job and losing out on the high-priority activity of being with your family.

Usually, a budget is balanced by the reallocation of expenditure. Look at the figures. Are you paying more for some things than you need to? Identify the low-priority items and start by cutting these. Are there some items of expenditure that give you a poor happiness return? Cut these too.

When you engage in cost-trimming, make sure your decisions are in keeping with your identified goals. If you have trouble with this, get some expert assistance (see p. 202).

Make your money go further

- *Plan ahead.* Don't wait until you have to purchase something in a hurry. Anticipate your needs so you can take advantage of special offers or at least shop around.
- *Use credit wisely.* A credit card can be useful — you can take advantage of an unexpected bargain, or obtain something you need when you don't have cash available — but make sure you are not tempted to make unnecessary purchases.
- *Avoid unnecessary financial costs.* Pay bills early when there is a discount offered for doing so. Pay credit card accounts in full by the due date to avoid incurring interest, which can be crippling. (If you need credit, use other, cheaper sources of finance, such as a bank loan or hire-purchase.) If using credit has been a problem for you in the past, train yourself to wait and save for items you don't need immediately.
- *Reduce the chance of overspending.* When shopping, don't take more money than you can afford to spend. If using a cheque book or credit card, set a limit and stay within it.
- *Plan your shopping trips.* Take a prepared list to the supermarket and stick to it. Resist additional items that take your fancy. Try to avoid taking children, or make it clear they are not to ask you to buy anything that isn't on the list. Go shopping once a week and get everything you need to save time and running expenses. Take a calculator and compare prices to see what package sizes are most economical.
- *Save money on holidays and recreation.* Camp rather than use motels. Sleep at home and make day trips to places of interest. Develop recreational activities and fun things to do at home with the family — board games, badminton in the backyard, barbecues (use sausages instead of steak, and pine cones, which are not only free but also give more flavour than a fancy, expensive, gas-operated cooker).
- *Eat well without breaking the bank.* Plan your meals a week in advance. Use grocery coupons and specials. Have some meals without meat. Keep fast foods to a minimum — they are expensive and low in nutritional value.
- *Shop around.* Check your insurance coverage to see if you can get a better deal elsewhere, get two or three quotes when your car tyres need replacing, and so on.
- *Buy in bulk* — providing the savings are significant and you can use all of what you buy.

- *Grow your own* fruit and vegetables if possible.
- *Learn how to preserve food,* and take advantage of good bulk buys or items you grow yourself (but check first the cost of any preserving materials).
- *Dress well for less.* Buy colour-coordinated clothing you can mix and match. Buy clothes you can wear through all seasons, adding or discarding layers as the weather changes. Buy on sale, but watch out for false economy; for example, don't buy clothes of poor quality or limited versatility. Avoid clothing that requires special and expensive care such as dry-cleaning. Modify an outfit you already own so that it looks and feels different. Add accessories to give something a new look. Take care of your wardrobe so it lasts and continues to look good.
- *Save money on maintenance.* Keep important maintenance up to date. Saving on oil changes is false economy when your car's engine wears out before its time. Delaying house painting may cost you extra in weather-damage repairs. Sometimes paying a little more will mean lower maintenance costs and longer life. On other occasions, a cheaper item will do the job just as well.

Overcoming the blocks to living within your means

Make sure your goals are clear

If you don't know what you really want out of life, sensible budget planning will be impossible, and you will be open to manipulation or impulse buying. The principles of *self-knowledge* (p. 54), *enlightened self-interest* (p. 58) and *self-direction* (p. 68) will help you here:

- Knowing your wants, aims and goals is the starting point to effective financial planning and rational buying decisions.
- Check that your spending benefits both yourself and those important to you. When tempted to buy something not part of your plan, ask yourself: 'Will buying this be in my interests?', 'Will it create problems for other key people in my life?', 'What am I prepared to forego to have it?', 'Will this work out with the other people in my life?'
- Make sure your spending decisions are based on what you really want out of life, not on 'shoulds' or the opinions of others.

199

Raise your tolerance for frustration and discomfort

Low frustration tolerance will lead you to seek short-term gratification rather than longer-term gains. It may make it hard to overcome inertia, stop drifting and start planning your life. You may watch television instead of painting the house, or procrastinate over paying your bills. The key principle here is *tolerance for frustration and discomfort* (p. 60):

- When changing your spending habits, resisting the impulse to buy or facing the discomfort of preparing a budget, remind yourself that the frustration you feel is unpleasant but not fatal.
- Apply *exposure* (p. 88) and *paradoxical behaviour* (p. 89). Practise tolerating frustration and discomfort. For a while, deliberately postpone any non-essential purchases. Schedule a time to start on that budget plan. Make appointments to see creditors you cannot pay right away.

Trust your judgement

If you don't trust your own judgement, you may end up letting others decide what is right for you, or avoid asking for information on products or services through fear others will think you ignorant. *Self-acceptance and confidence* (p. 55) will help you:

- If you accept yourself, you will have less need to buy things just to boost your ego or impress others. You will be less afraid to show your ignorance and ask for the information you need to make sensible spending decisions. And you will be able to make mistakes and learn from them without the fear of self-downing.
- With confidence will come a belief in your ability to make decisions. Sometimes it will be wise to collect information or seek the opinions of other people, but in the end, you will be best served by weighing the evidence and deciding what is best for you.

Keep your budgeting in proportion

Some people become obsessed with saving money. They travel long distances or search for weeks to find an item at a lower price than elsewhere. They spend hours repairing something which could be cheaply replaced. They fail to realise that time is valuable, too. What are your priority goals? To save money for its own sake, or to put your time into pleasurable and rewarding activities? Apply the principles of *moderation* (p. 65) and *flexibility* (p. 71):

- Cut back on extravagances when finances are tight, but also keep your money-saving activities in proportion. Don't become so obsessed that you forget the point of having money, which is to spend it in such a way as to attain your goals.
- Recognise the importance of adapting to changing circumstances, and be able to let go of some spending and consuming habits and replace them with others.

Don't buy just for emotional reasons

People frequently spend money not because they need what they buy, but for other, usually subconscious purposes, e.g. for revenge, to get attention or affection, to alleviate guilt, to lift a depressed mood, to boost their ego or to impress others. Unfortunately, money spent in this fashion is often wasted. Worse, energy is diverted from learning to deal with emotions in more productive ways. The principle of *long-range enjoyment* (p. 62) will help you here:

- Make a practice of planning all purchases in advance, postponing any that are inappropriate and only buying items that are on your list.
- Keep in mind the purpose of doing without something you want. It is not to make you a person of high moral calibre. The real purpose is more down-to-earth: to obtain greater pleasure later on. Don't forgo that new outfit because it would be 'wrong' to buy it; do so because you want to save for an overseas trip. This will be far more motivating.
- Most importantly, develop your ability to use *Rational Self-Analysis* (p. 80) and other *Rational Effectiveness* techniques (Chapter 8) as effective methods of dealing with unwanted emotions.

Resist compulsive or addictive spending

Some people feel compelled to buy things they don't really need without ensuring they have sufficient funds. This can range from the compulsive collection of unnecessary items at the expense of more important ones, to running up financially crippling credit accounts. This process may start as a way of alleviating bad feelings or compensating for something missing in life. As each spending episode makes the person feel temporarily better, an addiction is steadily cemented in place. Key principles that will help are *objective thinking* (p. 72), *emotional and behavioural responsibility* (p. 66) and *acceptance of reality* (p. 75):

- Don't see your finances as under the control of magical forces such as 'fate' or 'luck'. Take control of your own destiny.
- Ensure you are not making yourself a victim by blaming others — your children, partner, employer, the bank, the government — for your difficulties in managing money. Accepting responsibility for your own actions will help you take control.
- Recognise that the universe is not set up to provide everything you want. If you rid yourself of any demanding beliefs that you 'should' be able to have such-and-such, or that you absolutely 'need' it, you will find it easier to keep your spending and your life under control.
- Plan all purchases in advance and, when doing the shopping, stick to the list.
- Practise *postponing gratification* (p. 89); allow yourself some non-essentials, but delay their purchase.

Further training and help

Why not attend classes, workshops, seminars or other forms of training at which you can learn how to get more from your resources — healthy eating on a budget, do-it-yourself, and so on? Obtain other information from books or your local Citizens Advice Bureau.

Are you having trouble drawing up and sticking to a budget? Are you in so much debt you can't see your way out? Most communities have a Budget Advice Service which offers free advice.

Some problems will be resistant to self-help. Compulsive spending, gambling or alcohol and drug abuse can be addictions that are hard to break. Don't let these problems continue to wreck your life — get professional help. Try to find a counsellor or therapist who, rather than dig up your past, will help you discover and change whatever is keeping you addicted in the present, and show you how to stay free in the future.

Changing the myths about money

Self-defeating beliefs	Rational alternatives
Money is evil.	Money is a means of exchange. I can choose to become obsessed with it, or use it to achieve my goals.
I need money to be happy.	Money is relevant to security and health, but my emotions ultimately result from what I think rather than from what I have.

Self-defeating beliefs	*Rational alternatives*
I shouldn't need to budget my money.	Where is it written that I 'should' be exempt from what most of the human race does if it wants to get on?
I don't have enough money to budget.	I don't have enough money *not* to budget! The less you have, the more you need to plan what you do with it.
If I had more money, I would be more satisfied.	Expectations increase along with income! If I *prefer* to have more but avoid thinking I 'must', I will be satisfied enough to get on with life.

Further reading on financial management

Cash, Grady. *Conquer the Seven Deadly Money Mistakes.* Center for Financial Well-Being, Rancho Cordova, CA (Internet — http://www.ns.net/cash/), 1994.

Newman, Frank. *How to Live off the Smell of an Oily Rag.* Pursuit Publishing, Auckland, 1991.

Newman, Frank. *More Ways to Live off the Smell of an Oily Rag.* Oily Rag Books, Auckland, 1996.

18
Manage the Changes in Your Life

Chapter 15 explored the importance of stimulation and variety in life. Now it is time to look at the other side of the coin — how to cope when there is *too much* going on.

There is nothing new about change. Human beings have always passed through the various stages of the life cycle, adjusted to bonding with a mate and the arrival of children, reconciled themselves to the deaths of significant others and adapted to the ageing process. Such adjustments remain the lot of humans today.

What is new is the *pace* of change. Isaac Asimov has said that 'It is change, continuing change, inevitable change, that is the dominant factor in society today'.[1] Unfortunately, though, as James Baldwin is reported to have said: 'Most of us are about as eager to be changed as we were to be born, and go through our changes in a similar state of shock.'[2]

If both Asimov and Baldwin are correct, then we are faced with two conflicting facts of life. Humans generally dislike change, yet live in a world where change is inevitable. In fact it is apparent that the pace of change is accelerating.

The shock of change

Alvin Toffler graphically describes the problems of coping with change in his 1970 book *Future Shock*.[3] He explains how people can be psychologically overwhelmed when faced with disaster situations such as major earthquakes, tornadoes or tidal waves, in which homes are wrecked, loved ones killed and lives turned upside down. What is common to such situations is exposure to unfamiliar or unpredictable events and conditions. The senses are bombarded to such an extent they do not have time to recover from one stimulus before another occurs.

When there is too much change

As well as major disasters, everyday events can lead to a feeling of being overwhelmed when a number of changes occur close together. Three years before Toffler's book, Holmes and Rahe published 'The Social Readjustment Rating Scale',[4] which showed how people respond, in terms of their physical and emotional health, to common life events. Some of the items from this scale are reproduced below. The numbers indicate the level of stress associated with a given event, 100 being the highest:

Event	Rating	Event	Rating
Death of a spouse	100	Change in responsibilities at work	29
Marital separation	65	Son or daughter leaving home	29
Marriage	50	Outstanding achievement	28
Retirement	45	Trouble with boss or supervisor	23
Pregnancy	40	Change in residence	20
Gaining a new family member	39	Going on holiday	13
Major change in financial state	38	Christmas approaching	12
Change to a different line of work	36	Minor legal violations	11

You may be surprised to see events listed that most people would not regard as negative. This highlights an important point: even supposedly positive experiences can trigger some level of stress.

Note that the ratings are averages. Your own perception of an event may differ from that indicated by the rating given. Note too that the scale does not imply that events and circumstances themselves cause stress. What it shows is that people *perceive* certain events and circumstances in differing ways; and, as we have seen throughout this book, a person's perception of an event determines their reaction to it.

One or a few life events may not lead to significant distress. In fact, as already observed, some degree of challenge and stimulation is essential to good emotional health. But when a sufficient number of events perceived as distressful occur close in time, a person's coping system may become overloaded, as with these examples:

- A mid-level manager in a restructuring company is faced with multiple demands requiring complex decisions. Overload occurs when she has a minor motor-vehicle accident shortly after her daughter's wedding.

- A university student is faced with large amounts of information on a variety of subjects, a number of assignments, and examinations. He experiences overloading when ill health and problems with flatmates occur close together.
- A homemaker faces the demands of children, meal times, the telephone ringing and people calling at the door. The illness of a parent at the same time as the family is moving house leads to overload.

Why we need to adapt to change

The world is changing, and will go on changing. A major area of change, as Toffler explains in his book *Powershift*,[5] is the movement from an economy based on capital and manual labour to one based on knowledge and the use of skill. Applying knowledge and highly developed skills means the use of less labour, energy, capital, raw materials and time. But this carries a cost. If less physical labour is required while knowledge and skills grow in importance, individuals face a need to retrain and adapt to new ways of working.

Another key area of contemporary change is in the way people progress through the life cycle. As Gail Sheehy points out in *New Passages*,[6] people are taking longer to 'grow up' and longer to die. Consequently, the various stages of adulthood are moving backward by up to ten years. People are having their children later, those in their 40s, 50s and 60s feel five to ten years younger, men are increasingly forced into early retirement. These demographic changes require us to make corresponding changes in our attitudes toward, and preparation for, the various stages of ageing. Sheehy argues, for instance, that we can now see age forty-five as the beginning of a second adulthood.

If individuals (or societies) try to avoid change, it continues around them. They gradually become further out of touch and isolated from the wider environment. Sooner or later, the environment impacts on them in a way that cannot be ignored. Then the adjustment required may be major and disorienting.

At an individual level, you may know people who refuse to adapt and complain endlessly about how the world has gone, alienating themselves more and more. The same process can happen at a societal or national level. Albania, for instance, was isolated from the rest of the world by its paranoid dictator, Enver Hoxhar, who effectively denied his country any chance of participating in the technological advances of the second half of the twentieth century. Albania survived economically by taking hand-outs first from Russia then from China. When these dried up and the Communist regimes in surrounding countries were overthrown in the 1990s, the Albanian dictatorship eventually collapsed, leaving a poverty-ridden country economically on its knees, with little of the infrastructure taken for granted in the rest of Europe.

What this illustrates is that change, uncomfortable though it may be, is inevitable. Trying to ignore it brings short-term comfort at the expense of long-term pain.

Strategies to make change work for you

Given that change is often uncomfortable and stressful in the short term, what can you do to manage it? Fortunately, there are a number of strategies available.

Plan and prepare for change

You can often ease the impact of change by anticipating and preparing for it. Retirement, for example, is a time when finances reduce, health problems increase, housing needs alter and there is a substantial increase in spare time. If you save for retirement you can lessen the financial pain. Developing a regular fitness and healthy eating routine when younger can minimise health problems later. Moving to a smaller, low-maintenance property while still mobile will make it easier to establish relationships in the new locality. And developing fresh interests prior to retirement will prevent the boredom that can afflict people who suddenly find a lot of time on their hands, or for whom physical activities like work or sport have been the only source of stimulation in their lives.

Space changes

Try to anticipate changes and avoid too many major events close in time. Some occurrences, such as the death of a loved one, are unpredictable, but many can be anticipated and spaced. If a child is leaving home, you might delay changing your job. You could hold off major financial decisions soon after a bereavement; or postpone upgrading your car when you have just had surgery.

Minimise overstimulation

When you feel overloaded, try to follow familiar, comfortable routines until you get your energy back. Delegate or postpone decisions. Put off situations which involve meeting new people and temporarily stick with those you already know and feel comfortable with. Resist unnecessary changes in organisations to which you belong (while keeping in mind that progressive change and development may be required to avoid radical change later on).

Use support networks

Support groups (p. 222) can help with negotiating change. They bring together people going through a similar life transition — bereavement, unemployment, separation, new parenthood, retirement, etc. Such groups are not for 'therapy', but for support and mutual help in clarifying goals and sharing strategies for managing the transition. Involvement in a group is only for as long as it takes the individual to adjust.

Counselling (p. 223) is another form of support. Redundancy, separation and retirement counselling are examples of how people can be helped to deal with change in a structured way.

Maintain personal stability zones

We can cope more effectively with change by maintaining what Toffler calls 'personal stability zones'.[7] Here are some examples:

- *Retain comfortable and valued elements of your physical environment.* Keep clothes for longer — resist new fashion trends. Keep your car for longer — avoid changing it for the sake of minor enhancements. Don't upgrade computer software every time a new version comes out. Keep furniture if it is comfortable and suitable for its purpose; have it reconditioned rather than replaced.
- *Maintain some old friends and acquaintances* with whom you feel comfortable, even as you meet new people. Be open to fresh experiences, new literature, new music — but have favourite things to fall back on when you need a bit less stimulation.
- *Maintain any daily habits that are usually functional for you* even when you are out of your normal environment. For example, when travelling, endeavour to go to bed and get up at your usual times, have your daily relaxation period, read before going to bed as normal, or do whatever it is your habit to do.
- *Maintain rituals that provide continuity* in the face of change. As Imber-Black and Roberts explain in their book *Rituals for Our Times*,[8] rituals have the capacity to ease difficult life transitions by providing a sense of connection with others and with the past. Many people, though, have become isolated from the rituals they were brought up with

owing to factors like migration, remarriage or the separation of parents. There may be a need to develop new rituals that are more appropriate and meaningful to the present. There can be rituals around daily events like bedtimes, leaving and returning home, leisure activities and weekends, as well as special occasions such as birthdays, relationship anniversaries, reunions and starting or leaving school. All contribute to a sense of continuity, even when the rituals themselves alter to reflect individual and family changes.

Have more than one source of satisfaction in your life

The more connections you have with the world at large — family, friends, coworkers, church, clubs — the more sources of support you can call on to help manage the stress of change.

These connections, along with your various hobbies and other interests, will also be the sources of satisfaction and enjoyment in your life. Having multiple sources of satisfaction can be helpful when one area of your life is not going well. You may compensate for stressful changes at work, for example, by continuing to get enjoyment from your children, social activities and other pursuits.

Keep your reactions in proportion

Finally, and most importantly, keep your emotional reactions in proportion to the changes you are facing. If you have been made redundant, be concerned rather than fearful. When your child is leaving home, feel sad but not depressed. When there are more things to do than time available, be alert but not tense. Use the strategies of *Rational Effectiveness Training* (Chapter 8) to identify and change the self-defeating thinking that underlies any dysfunctional emotions or behaviours.

Overcoming the blocks to managing change

Be able to assert yourself

Managing change will be difficult if you find it hard to say no or ask for what you want. If, say, your boss wants to schedule a major project when your daughter plans to have her wedding, you will have trouble negotiating if you are afraid to speak up. *Enlightened self-interest* (p. 58) will help:

- Tell other people when their plans conflict with yours, and negotiate changes to reduce the number of things that happen close together.

- Be prepared to alter your own plans when appropriate, at other times ask others to alter theirs.

Raise your discomfort tolerance

Are you prone to viewing some changes as 'awful' and 'unbearable'? Catastrophising about the badness of change will turn concern into anxiety and make you want to avoid or resist it. Established patterns of behaviour provide a sense of comfort and security, which change disrupts. You will find it hard to adapt if you have a low tolerance for discomfort. Apply the principles of *tolerance for discomfort* (p. 60), *long-range enjoyment* (p. 62), *risk-taking* (p. 64) and *moderation* (p. 65):

- Don't resist change or, at the other extreme, be passive about it: actively embrace it. This will be easier when you see change as uncomfortable but not unbearable.
- Change is often easier to bear if it is viewed in a long-term perspective. *Time projection* (p. 88) can help with this.
- Many changes contain an element of risk. Remind yourself that calculated risks are an important part of achieving a stimulating and satisfying life, whereas avoidance of risk is a guarantee of boredom.
- Keep risk-taking in proportion by managing the change in your life. Spacing change and avoiding unnecessary change are ways of making it a positive rather than negative experience.

Be able to tolerate frustration

Low frustration tolerance arises from believing that certain events and circumstances 'should' or 'must not' occur. Do you hold any beliefs like: 'The balance of my life must not be disturbed', or 'I shouldn't have to make adjustments'? Ideas like these will exacerbate anxiety and lead to anger or feelings of hopelessness. Key principles here are *tolerance for frustration* (p. 60), *emotional and behavioural responsibility* (p. 66) and *flexibility* (p. 71):

- Dispute any idea you may have that you personally should be exempt from change. See the frustrations involved with change as something to grow with, not a burden to be avoided.
- Take responsibility for how you feel and behave, instead of blaming it on other people, the government or fate. This will give you more motivation to influence change, and help you handle your feelings when change does not go the way you want.

- Developing flexibility as a guiding principle in your life will guard against blind resistance or avoidance. It will help you adapt, to bend with the storm rather than be broken by it.

Accept change

Non-acceptance of change can show in many ways. Some people, for example, have trouble accepting the ageing process. A woman anxious about physical attractiveness may engage in dangerous dieting as ageing leads to normal weight increase. An older man overconcerned with physical performance may run the risk of injury by continuing to play contact sports. You can help yourself accept change with the principles of *self-acceptance* (p. 55), *objective thinking* (p. 72), *self-direction* (p. 68) and *acceptance of reality* (p. 75):

- Work on accepting yourself irrespective of your changing appearance or abilities. Enjoy being an older person instead of denying the reality of passing youth. Focus on maximising the quality of your life now, rather than trying to relive the past.
- Rid yourself of any notion that change is the result of 'fate' or unspecified supernatural forces and therefore you can't do anything about it.
- When change is in the air, don't deny or avoid it — get involved. Join the committee set up to implement reorganisation at work. Get to know your local Member of Parliament and express your views. Write to newspapers. Start a neighbourhood action group. Use your energy not to avoid change but to influence it in a productive direction. Sometimes it will be in your interests to *initiate* change rather than just respond to it. If you are bored with your job, don't complain; ask for fresh tasks or responsibilities, or consider a new job or even a change of career. If there are inefficiencies at work, don't wait for others to put them right; initiate the appropriate measures yourself.
- Some changes will be negative experiences for you, and out of your control. Where you do have a choice, though, is in how you react to them. Either you can rail against fate and spend the rest of your life consumed with bitterness. Or you can choose to grieve for your loss, pick yourself up and get on with life. Don't resist change, or ignore it. As Aldous Huxley wrote in his *Collected Essays*: 'Enlightenment is not for the quietists and puritans who, in their different ways, deny the world, but for those who have learned to accept and transfigure it.'

Changing your beliefs about change

Self-defeating beliefs	Rational alternatives
The world is getting worse.	Some things are getting worse, some things are getting better.
I can't stand to have my life disrupted.	I dislike disruption, but obviously I can stand it; it's happened many times and I'm still alive to tell the tale!
Life should be predictable and certain.	Life has never been predictable and certain. Where is it written that it 'should' be so now?
It would be selfish to ask others to change their plans when they conflict with mine.	It is enlightened to take into account the wishes of others; self-*interested* (rather than self*ish*) to do the same with mine.
It is easier to avoid change and its attendant discomfort and pain.	It is (sometimes) easier in the short term to avoid change, but to do so makes it harder later on.
I can't help feeling bad in response to the changes in my life.	How I feel in response to change depends on what I tell myself about it. And I can have control over my beliefs.
What will happen will happen, so you can't influence change.	If I believe this, I will most probably end up fulfilling my own prophecy!
To be unchanging shows stability and strength.	Resisting change demonstrates anxiety and rigidity. Working with and influencing change shows courage and flexibility.

Further reading on managing change

Imber-Black, Evan, and Roberts, Janine. *Rituals for Our Times*. Harper Perennial, New York, 1992.

Sheehy, Gail. *New Passages: Mapping your life across time*. HarperCollins Publishers, London, 1996.

Toffler, Alvin. *Future Shock*. Pan Books, London, 1970.

Toffler, Alvin. *Powershift: Knowledge, Wealth, and Violence at the Edge of the 21st Century*. Bantam Books, New York, 1990.

19
Know How to Problem-Solve

We engage in problem-solving many times a day. Much of the time we do it unawares, at other times we consciously grapple with a problem. Choosing an ice-cream flavour, balancing a budget and finding care for an elderly parent are all examples of problem-solving.

Problem-solving is required in all areas of life, from dealing with emergency situations to choosing which brand of tinned tomatoes to buy. Your problem-solving skills come from many sources, including the knowledge you gather from experience or formal learning, your ability to think and reason, and your capacity for emotional self-control.

How does problem-solving relate to stress management? While it is true that distress results from how we view things rather than from problems themselves, if we can reduce the impact of these on our lives and get more of what we want (and less of what we don't), so much the better.

The problem-solving process

Sometimes a problem is difficult to solve, and calls for a structured approach. This involves going through a series of steps: defining the problem, getting information, developing courses of action, putting these into practice and evaluating the results.

In my previous book, *Choose to be Happy*, I describe such a problem-solving process in detail.[1] What follows is a summary, with minor variations, of that process. It is one you can use when you have problems that require major decisions, or when there is no obvious course of action.

You don't have to go through all the stages with every problem. Some issues can be dealt with quickly. Others, especially those that involve major changes in your life, could warrant spreading the process over days or even weeks.

When faced with a difficult problem — stop! Don't panic and do the first thing that comes to mind. If your emotions are running high, free up your thinking by doing a *Rational Self-Analysis* (p. 80).

Step 1: Spell out the problem
State the problem in concrete terms. Be specific: 'Our average weekly expenditure is $180.00 more than our income' is better than 'We can't make ends meet.' Also, break the problem down into its various parts. This will help you see it more clearly and work on it in small chunks. Be very clear as to exactly what it is you see as problematic.

Step 2: Collect information
Gather information on the problem. There are some tips on doing this later (p. 217).

Step 3: Set goals
Express the various parts of the problem as goals. State these as specifically as possible so you can know when they have been achieved. 'Be able to keep our spending within our income and save $2,000.00 per year' is a goal that can be objectively measured.

Don't settle on your final goals until you have considered everything you might wish for, however fanciful. 'I wish our creditors would all disappear' may be asking for the unlikely, but it might trigger some creative thinking that could lead to: 'Maybe we could get rid of our creditors by increasing our mortgage.'

Step 4: Develop alternative strategies
First, list a range of possible strategies for reaching the goals you have set. Use the brainstorming procedure — that is, write down every potential solution you can think of, no matter how way-out any of them may seem. The idea is to generate the largest number of options you can. Don't criticise any or attempt to analyse how workable they are. At this stage, go for quantity rather than quality. 'Go busking for money' deserves a place alongside 'Draw up a budget.' Even highly impractical ideas may serve to trigger other, more realistic ones.

Next, decide which strategies to pursue. Carefully examine all the options you have written down. Ask three key questions about each:

1. What are the likely *consequences* of pursuing this — both negative and positive, for myself and significant others, in both the long and short term?
2. How does this fit with my *personal value system*?
3. How *useful* would this be in helping me achieve the goal I have set?

(This is where you decide that busking is out because you can't sing very well.)

A single strategy may be enough to achieve a goal, or you may need to follow several courses of action before you get there. Sometimes there will not be any solution that is desirable; the best you can do then is decide which would be the least unsatisfactory option.

Step 5: Identify any blocks to your strategies

Is there anything which might prevent you from applying the strategies you have chosen? Identify it now. For example, if your children are used to an allowance you can no longer afford, think about ways to get them to cooperate with the new financial regime.

Step 6: Develop tactics

By now you will have decided on one or more strategies aimed at achieving your various goals. You could describe these stategies as *sub-goals*. Now it is time to generate some *tactics* — that is, specific actions for carrying out your strategies (and so achieving your sub-goals). Tactics are what you actually *do*.

Let's say, for example, that your strategy is 'Get budgeting help.' Some tactics might be:

1. Ring Citizens Advice Bureau to see what budgeting organisations exist in our area.
2. Talk to some friends who have had budgeting help.

Once again, use the brainstorming method described in Step 3. Go for the maximum number of ideas. You might consider such activities as consulting the local budgeting service, obtaining a library book or consumers' magazine about saving household costs, or talking to your creditors.

Next, select the tactics to put into action. Be guided in your selection by asking the same questions as at Step 4. What are the likely consequences of each tactic? How does it fit with my personal value system? Will it be useful in implementing the strategy concerned? Also ask: Will this tactic get around the potential blocks I have identified?

Step 7: Put your tactics into action

Carry out the tactics you have chosen.

Step 8: Evaluate the results

If you do not obtain the results you desire, don't give up. Return to an earlier stage of the process and start again from there.

How to make decisions

An important part of problem-solving is deciding between alternatives. What follows is a technique that provides a structure for what may otherwise seem a daunting process.

On a sheet of paper, draw a chart like the one below. (Include columns for further options if you wish.) Under each option, list its advantages and disadvantages. Give each of these a rating according to how important it is to you: 1 for the least important, 10 for the most. Calculate a total for each option by adding up the advantages ratings and subtracting the disadvantages ratings.

	Option 1 *Go bankrupt*	Weight	Option 2 *Get budgeting help*	Weight
Advantages	Would wipe out all debts so could make a fresh start.	9	Would repay all debts, even though slowly.	9
	No more pressure from creditors.	8	Would learn how to manage money and stay out of debt.	10
Disadvantages	Wouldn't be able to leave country.	2	Would take a long time to repay debts.	7
	Would be barred from starting another business.	7	Would have to expose incompetence with money to others.	6
	Creditors would never get paid, which hard for some of them.	8		
	Wouldn't learn anything about handling money.	9		
	Total	**–9**	**Total**	**+6**

Note that advantages and disadvantages include consequences that are both *practical* (e.g. Would learn how to manage money) and *emotional* (e.g. Would have to expose incompetence).

Totalling each column of ratings and comparing the results will help you decide which option to take, although sometimes it is a good idea to look beyond the figures and consider how you feel about each option at a gut level. If your intuition tells you something different from what the numbers say, ask yourself if you have been entirely honest in all your ratings.

Some problem-solving suggestions

When there is more than one problem

It is usually best to deal with problems in order of needs first, then desires. Satisfaction of a higher-level *desire* is unlikely when lower-level *needs* remain unmet. Social desires or aspirations, for instance, are not likely to be an issue when you lack food. Developing a talent will usually take second place to finding somewhere to live. The following chart, which I have adapted from the hierarchy of needs described by psychologist Abraham Maslow,[2] illustrates the progression from needs to desires:

Desires

Self-actualisation	Self-fulfilment through developing talents, abilities and potential
Positive view of self	Self-respect, a sense of competence
Social connection	Feeling of belonging, receiving affection, intimacy
Safety and security	Shelter, avoidance of pain
Physical survival	Food, water, rest

Necessities

Trying to solve more than one problem at a time may leave you feeling overwhelmed. If you pick off your problems one by one, you will have a much better chance of dealing with them effectively. Separate and prioritise them so the most important get dealt with first. If you are concerned you might forget any, make a record of those you are putting on hold.

Getting information to aid problem-solving

To develop effective solutions you require information. Here is a process to help you gather information relevant to a problem you are working on:

- *Identify what information you need.* After you have defined the problem, ask: 'What do I need to know to reach a solution?'
- *Identify possible sources of information* — your own experience, other

people, community education classes, organisations, books, maga-zines, audio- or video-tapes, the Internet, etc.

- *Access the sources you have identified.*
- *Extract the information.* Be selective; try to record only relevant infor-mation, and summarise it so you are not overwhelmed by facts.
- *Synthesise the information.* Put together the separate pieces of infor-mation to form a new combination that addresses the problem.

Practise on less critical problems

Don't wait for a really big problem to arise before you learn to problem-solve — practise on less critical difficulties. See how the above method works for you; modify it to suit your individual style.

Overcoming the blocks to solving problems

Make sure you are internally directed

If you believe your life is under the control of external forces, you may see little point in trying to change anything. You can help yourself with the principles of *objective thinking* (p. 71), *emotional and behavioural responsi-bility* (p. 66) and *self-direction* (p. 68):

- Give up any 'magical' thinking that leads you to put your head in the sand and rely on mystical forces such as 'fate' to direct your life.
- No matter what the cause of a problem, keep in mind that you are responsible for what you do about it. This will help you move from blaming to solving. Also, by taking responsibility for how you feel, you can avoid upsetting yourself more than you need to.
- Don't see yourself as a victim. Rather than sit around blaming or waiting to be rescued, start looking at possible solutions. Use others for advice and support, but in the end make your own decisions on what is to be done. Except when there is good reason to have some-one else do it, action those decisions yourself.

Be clear about your values

If decisions and solutions are to be right for you, they need to be in line with your values. *Self-knowledge* (p. 54) is the key:

- Identifying your goals and values will help you make decisions you can live with. See Chapter 9 if you need help with this.

Separate 'shoulds' from wants

You will have trouble making decisions when there is a conflict between what you *want* to do and what you think you 'should' do. A want won't go away even if a 'should' is demanding your compliance. Use the principle of *enlightened self-interest* (p. 58) to break through the 'shoulds':

- Judge potential solutions according to how they serve your interests, but also take into account how they affect other people.

Avoid perfectionism

Black-and-white thinking and demanding could lead you to believe that decisions and solutions are either completely 'right' or completely 'wrong', and that you must always find the 'right' one. However, because there is no such thing as a perfect solution, your demand for one could paralyse you from doing anything at all. You can help yourself by practising the principle of *flexibility* (p.71):

- Keep in mind that there are no black or white answers.
- Judge potential solutions according to their degree of usefulness, not 'rightness'.
- Be open to a range of options. In a rapidly changing world, it is necessary to look beyond old solutions.

Tolerate discomfort and frustration

To weigh one thing against another creates internal conflict. You may be tempted to avoid this discomfort by putting off decisions or actions. There are risks involved in committing yourself to a course of action and carrying it out; you might start something you can't finish, or events could turn out badly. Accordingly, you may choose the 'safe' path of avoidance. Also, to decide on one option means letting go of others. Low frustration tolerance may lead you to hold onto all the options and thus choose none. Four principles can be applied here — *tolerance for frustration and discomfort* (p. 60), *long-range enjoyment* (p. 62), *risk-taking* (p. 64) and *acceptance of reality* (p. 75):

- Challenge the idea that you should be able to lead a life free of problems and not have to make difficult decisions or carry out uncomfortable actions. When you expect frustration and discomfort, paradoxically, they become easier to handle.

- Ensure that your problem-solving takes account of your long-term interests rather than simply providing short-term relief. With each option, consider whether it will make things better or worse in the long run.
- Accept that making decisions and acting on them usually involves some risk. Ask yourself: 'Is the risk of doing the wrong thing as harmful to my interests as doing nothing?'
- There will always be some problems that cannot be resolved. If you change what you can and accept what you can't, you will avoid paralysing yourself with bitterness or hopelessness.

Accept yourself

If you connect your 'self-worth' with doing things 'right' and never making mistakes, you will be tempted to avoid action because your self-image will be on the line. If you worry that other people will disapprove of what you do, you will be even less likely to get into action. And if you regard yourself as less important than others, you are likely to keep putting their interests ahead of your own. Use the principles of *self-acceptance* (p. 55) and *enlightened self-interest* (p. 58):

- Give up the idea that you have to be a 'worthwhile' human being, and that 'worthwhileness' depends on your performance and getting approval from others.
- Ask yourself how it is that the interests of others are more important than your own.

Have confidence in your own judgment

If you don't trust yourself or your opinions, you are likely to become paralysed when trying to decide what to do, or leave it to others to decide for you. *Confidence* (p. 55) and *risk-taking* (p. 64) are the keys:

- Seek opinions from other people, but in the end make up your own mind about what is best for you.
- Acknowledge that nothing is guaranteed, and that taking calculated risks is essential to getting anywhere.
- Do a *benefits calculation* (p. 86) to check out the risks and benefits of particular options.

Further reading on problem-solving

Froggatt, Wayne. *Choose to be Happy: Your step-by-step guide.* HarperCollins Publishers, Auckland, 1993.

20
Ask for Help When You Need It

This book has presented a range of skills for use in minimising unhealthy reactions to stress. Most of them you will be able to learn and use on yourself throughout your life. However, from time to time, like most other people, you may face situations that are unfamiliar and beyond your experience. These are the times at which it makes sense to ask for help.

Where you can get help

Help can range from informal support given by a friend or neighbour, to professional help with a major difficulty.

Informal support

Most support comes from informal sources like partners, relatives, friends, neighbours and coworkers. It may involve nothing more than a listening ear from a neighbour or advice from a colleague during a coffee break.

Support groups

These are groups in which people get together with others who have a similar problem, to share support and advice. Here are some examples of support groups which address specific problems:

- *Addiction:* SMART Recovery, Alcoholics Anonymous
- *Mental health:* Schizophrenia Fellowship, GROW, Phobic Trust
- *Physical illness or disability:* Cancer Society, Head Injury Support Group
- *Family problems:* Parentline, ToughLove
- *Negotiating life transitions:* Bereavement groups, Daycentres for the elderly

Self-help groups that are well run can be very effective. There is potential, though, for making a problem worse. This can happen when the focus is on whining about a problem rather than dealing with it. Such groups seek to turn members into 'victims', constantly complaining about injustices done and hindering any attempt to rise above their problems. Fortunately, most support groups are not like this, but always check out a group you are thinking of joining to ensure it is devoted either to developing solutions, or to helping people reach acceptance. Talk to others who have had involvement with the group, or attend a trial session, before making up your mind.

Skills training

Skills training is designed to develop ability in areas such as assertiveness and communication. It can be obtained from an individual counsellor, although it is more usual to do such training in small groups. These are often provided by polytechnics, adult education classes or social service organisations.

Professional help

Sometimes, because of the difficulty or complexity of a problem, professional help is required.

- *Counselling* involves giving advice and assisting with decision-making and problem-solving, and may include skills training. It does not assume that the individual needs to change; instead, it attempts to find solutions to problems.
- *Psychotherapy* assumes that the problem lies mainly within the person, and seeks to help an individual make long-term changes in their typical ways of reacting to life. Psychotherapy is especially useful with emotional difficulties such as depression and anxiety, and in helping people change dysfunctional behaviours like addiction and violence.

In practice, counselling and psychotherapy are carried out together. Counselling often results in permanent change in an individual, and psychotherapy frequently needs to be combined with advice-giving or problem-solving.

Traditionally, counselling and psychotherapy have been provided by helping professionals such as psychologists and social workers, but in recent times training courses devoted specifically to counselling or psychotherapy have been available. Do not worry too much about the label a particular helping professional has. Instead, go on recommendations from an adviser you trust or someone who has actually consulted the professional concerned. Here are some of the more common sources of professional help:

- family doctor
- health service social worker or psychologist
- private counsellor/psychotherapist
- Maori health service.
- Marriage Guidance
- alcohol or drug addiction centre
- church social service

Support and crisis services

Sometimes there will be a problem that requires immediate help. Support in a crisis situation can be obtained from services such as Victim Support, Womens Refuge, Rape Crisis and the Lifeline telephone counselling service.

Where to get advice on sources of help

If you are unsure where to go for help, consider consulting your family doctor, pastor or local Citizens Advice Bureau, or other services advertised in your phone book.

Before you see a counsellor

You will increase the chance that counselling or psychotherapy will be a satisfying experience if you do some advance checking and monitor your ongoing contact with the counsellor. The following suggestions are drawn from the checklist developed by Stephen Palmer and Kasia Szymanska,[1] as well as from my own experience.

Questions to consider in advance or soon after commencing

- Does the counsellor have relevant qualifications and experience?
- Does the counsellor receive supervision from another professional counsellor or supervision group? (Most professional bodies consider supervision to be mandatory.)

- Is the counsellor a member of a professional body that has a clear code of ethics? (Obtain a copy of the code if possible.)
- What type of approach does the counsellor use and how does it relate to your problem?
- Discuss with the counsellor your goals and what you expect to get from the counselling.
- Ask about fees, if any, and discuss the frequency and estimated duration of your counselling.
- Finally, do not enter into a long-term counselling contract unless you are satisfied this is *necessary* and will be *beneficial* to you. (If in doubt, get a second opinion.)

Points to keep in mind when seeing a counsellor

- *Regular reviews.* Ask for periodic evaluations of progress toward your specified goals.
- *Keep the focus on your problems.* Self-disclosure by the counsellor can sometimes be therapeutically useful, but speak up if the sessions are dominated by the counsellor discussing his or her own problems.
- *Maintain appropriate boundaries between yourself and your counsellor.* Do not accept significant gifts (apart from relevant therapeutic material, such as reading) or social invitations (unless they are part of the therapeutic work itself — for instance, facing social anxiety by going with your counsellor to a crowded coffee bar). If your counsellor proposes a change in venue for your sessions — for example, from a centre to his or her own home — without good reason, do not agree. It is not beneficial (in fact, usually damaging) for clients to have sexual contact with their counsellor, and it is unethical for counsellors or therapists to engage in any such contact with their clients.
- *Express any concerns.* If at any time you feel discounted, undermined or manipulated, or have any doubts about the counselling you are receiving, discuss this with your counsellor. Try to resolve issues as they arise rather than sit on them. If you are still uncertain, seek advice. Talk to a friend, your doctor, your local Citizens Advice Bureau, the professional body to which your counsellor belongs, or the agency, if any, that employs him or her.

Overcoming the blocks to asking for help

Know that change is possible

If you don't see much chance of anything changing, you will let things drift. Use the principle of *objective thinking* (p. 72) to overcome inertia:

- Challenge any myths about accepting help, such as: 'No-one could help me unless they too have been through what I've experienced', or 'My problems are caused by events in my past, so little can be done to change them.' How do you know that change is impossible until you have given it a try?
- Dispute any 'magical' thinking that your emotions are controlled, or your life mapped out, by external forces.

Accepting help does not mean dependence

Do you believe people shouldn't need help with personal problems and should be able to 'stand on their own feet', or that to accept help would somehow be proof of 'weakness'? Do you worry that if you seek help from other people you will become dependent on them? Help yourself with the principles of *self-acceptance and confidence* (p. 55), *self-knowledge* (p. 54) and *emotional and behavioural responsibility* (p. 66):

- Accepting help does not prove you are a 'weak person'; all it proves is that you are a person who sometimes requires assistance.
- Trust your own judgements about the advice you get; decide which parts are right for you, and leave the rest.
- Know what your limits are. Know how far you can go with helping yourself, and when it is time to turn to other people for support and guidance.
- Remember that you create your own emotions and behaviours, and only you can change them. Other people can show you what to do, but only you can actually do it. If you keep this in mind, you are unlikely to become dependent.

You can stay in control

Do you worry that you will be made to do things against your will, such as taking medication, entering a psychiatric facility or adopting beliefs which are contrary to your values? Apply the principle of *self-direction* (p. 68):

- Take from others what will work for you and ignore the rest.
- If you sense a helper is trying to force something on you, discuss it with them. If they don't listen, exercise your choice to go elsewhere.

Confront fears about revealing yourself to others

Do you fear that a counsellor will regard you as insane, or that you will end up with a formal psychiatric diagnosis? Do you think that if you expose your thoughts and feelings to another person they will use what they learn to harm you or get power over you, or at the very least will look down on you? *Risk-taking* (p. 64) and *self-acceptance* (p. 55) are key principles for overcoming these fears:

- There are risks in accepting help. Sometimes people do make inappropriate use of what they learn; sometimes they do look down on others. But keep in mind three questions: Just how damaging would these things be if they did happen? How likely are they to happen? And is the risk worth it, bearing in mind the potential gain (or the certainty of staying where you are if you do nothing?).
- As you move from self-evaluation to self-acceptance, you will become less concerned about what others may think when you expose your thoughts and feelings to them.

Overcome the fear of changing

Most people would not consciously resist improving their condition, but sometimes there are secondary gains to be had from not changing. Getting attention through being ill is an example. The main motivation for not effecting change is probably the desire to avoid responsibility. If a person learns to handle stress, they remove a useful justification for avoiding life's problems, difficulties and challenges. Key principles here are *tolerance for frustration and discomfort* (p. 60) and *flexibility* (p. 71):

- If you accept discomfort as a normal part of life and believe that facing it is in your interests, you will feel easier about seeking help and beginning the process of personal change.
- Be open to exploring new ways of looking at yourself, others, the world and life in general. Opening up new vistas of opportunity and helping people change is the essence of counselling and psychotherapy.

Be realistic about change

Finally, watch out for any internal demand that you be able to change anything and everything you dislike. This may lead to potentially dangerous behaviour (such as radical dieting) and, finally, to disillusionment. The principle of *acceptance of reality* (p. 75) will help you avoid these dangers while still working hard at change:

- Go for help with optimism and a determination to achieve the change you want.
- But keep in mind that you can't change everything.
- How do you adopt this dual approach? Desire change, but hold your desire as a preference, not a demand.

Further reading on using help

Seligman, Martin E.P. *What You Can Change and What You Can't: The complete guide to successful self-improvement.* Random House, Sydney, 1994.

Pilpel, Robert H. *Understanding Your Therapist or Why is this taking so long?* Contemporary Books, Chicago, 1989.

Johnson, Catherine. *When to Say Goodbye to Your Therapist.* Simon and Schuster, New York, 1988.

21
Finale: Goodstress at Work

The principles in this book, as well as helping at a personal level, can be used to increase organisational effectiveness. The application of goodstress principles in the workplace warrants a book of its own, but this chapter will summarise some key aspects.

It begins by examining a type of stress that is particularly associated with work. Then several of the practical strategies described in Part Three are selected and their application in the workplace is demonstrated (although, of course, all the strategies can be applied in that context). A brief review follows of some of the many ways in which Rational Effectiveness Training can be used in the workplace. Finally, the chapter takes a look at how the Twelve Rational Principles can help workers and organisations not only cope, but also become more effective.

Burnout

There is a type of stress which, although it can occur in any situation, has been mainly documented in relation to the workplace.[1] Called *burnout,* it is the result of continued and unrelieved stress over a long period.

The typical symptoms are exhaustion, decline in job satisfaction, difficulty coping with role demands, absenteeism, impatience and bad temper, resentment toward colleagues and consumers, and alcohol abuse. It usually progresses in three stages.

How to identify burnout

In the *early stage,* the person affected may become overresponsible toward consumers and overinvolved with the job (staying late, not taking any breaks, avoiding colleagues), and experience minor health problems like colds and headaches.

In the *middle stage* there tends to be a continuous negative attitude towards the organisation accompanied by non-constructive complaining to coworkers and blaming of others, occasional inefficiency (through being slow, rude or forgetful), overcompliance, rigid application of rules and instructions, and worsening physical symptoms such as migraines, influenza, menstrual problems and backache.

In the *final stage,* there can be open conflict with the organisation featuring tears, rage, hearings, sacking or resignation; an inability to function in the work role leading to total retreat or paralysis; and more serious physical symptoms like nausea, anxiety and stomach problems, such that employment may be terminated for medical reasons. Psychiatric referral may follow. The person may renounce their profession or role and retreat to menial tasks or manual work.

Avoiding burnout

Recognising the early signs of burnout will allow you to take corrective action. Prevention, though, is better than cure: if you practise healthy living and good stress management, as described in this book, you will stay well away from even the early stages of burnout.

Getting support at work

Maintaining good relationships with others in the workplace is a key way to avoid burnout. It allows you to get help with problem-solving, avoid feelings of alienation and operate better as part of a team.

What causes isolation in the workplace?

- *Time.* If the workplace is busy, maintaining relationships may seem a low priority. People moving up the promotional ladder are especially prone to becoming 'too busy' to take time out to give and receive support.
- *Differences in status and power.* If you are in authority over someone, then you have more power than that person. Employees are only too aware a superior can recommend for or against their promotion; enhance or diminish their work satisfaction; and, ultimately, play a part in terminating their employment. This power differential makes it hard (and, mostly, undesirable) for managers to seek personal support from their subordinates.
- *Few peers available.* If you are in an executive position, there may be few people at your level easily available to you. This will become progressively worse as you move further up the ladder. Any compe-

tition among peers will make mutual support even more unlikely.

- *The assumption that support should 'just happen'.* People in the workplace often assume that integration into a group, and the giving and taking of support, are things that naturally happen. Consequently, they may do little to see that a new person is included and not take notice when a colleague begins to isolate him- or herself.

Make time!

It is incorrect to say we 'don't have time'. We always have time — twenty-four hours a day of it, seven days a week, fifty-two weeks a year. We use that time for whatever we regard as important.

You can choose to consider support in the workplace as a priority and allocate time to it. In fact, time spent on support is time well spent. Reducing stress increases efficiency and effectiveness.

Allow time for informal visiting and chatting with peers and subordinates. Linger behind after a meeting with a colleague. Talk to coworkers during your breaks and take other opportunities to socialise with them.

Look for support in many places

As well as informal contact, consider holding formal meetings with coworkers about your own or shared concerns. Arrange a regular time with a supervisor or mentor when you can deal with issues on a continuing basis. Take opportunities to meet people in your field from other workplaces, at conferences, seminars, workshops or interest-group meetings.

Return the favour

You can increase the likelihood of receiving support from others if you offer them support. The principle of *enlightened self-interest* (p. 58) is just as relevant to the workplace as it is to your personal life.

Maintain appropriate boundaries

If you are a manager or supervisor, communication with subordinates can help ease any sense of isolation you may be feeling, but it is important to maintain some boundaries. It may be appropriate to problem-solve with subordinates on work-related matters, but not to seek their help with your own emotional issues. Save these for your peers, partner or non-work friends.

Be wary of developing intimate relationships at work. Between peers, there may be some advantages: coworkers are easy to meet, you can learn about

231

them before committing yourself, and they are likely to be similar in socio-economic status, education and income level. But there are some dangers:[2]

- An attempt to start a romance may be construed as sexual harass-ment, even if one party thinks they are receiving encouragement from the other. Charges of sexual harassment are more likely when there is inequality in status and power between the people concerned.
- A proportion of workplace romances are extramarital affairs, which creates stress both in and out of the workplace.
- A romantic connection between manager and subordinate can be dangerous to both parties. Because of the power differential, it will not be an equal relationship. Coworkers may become jealous. If the relationship ends, one of the parties may have to leave the workplace.

If a supportive relationship at work develops into something more, stand back and ask: is this in my interests, or would I do better to re-establish the boundary?

Cultivate feedback

An important aspect of support at work is feedback on one's personal per-formance. Unfortunately, it is not easy to get honest feedback; people tend to be anxious to please and afraid to offend.

Directly invite people to be honest with you. When they give you nega-tive feedback, don't get defensive; encourage them to continue. Ask ques-tions. Help them clarify their thoughts and be specific in their comments.

You may find people within your organisation — a supervisor, mentor, or trusted colleague — who will provide you with honest feedback. It may also be appropriate, sometimes even necessary, to go outside the organis-ation and seek feedback from a spouse, friend or independent consultant.

To get started, complete a variation of the form illustrated on page 151. List your various areas of responsibility at work, then note potential sources of both support and feedback for each.

Assertiveness at work

Stuart Schmidt and David Kipnis[3] describe six strategies that people com-monly use to influence their superiors: reasoning, confrontation, friendli-ness, obtaining support from others, gaining the patronage of higher authorities, and bargaining.

Which work best? It appears that people who use confrontation, both men and women, end up with less than those who use reasoning and the other methods. Confronters also experience the highest levels of stress and the lowest levels of job satisfaction.

Many people confuse influence with power. But as Elaina Zuker[4] points out, power (in the sense of domination) is often the least effective form of influence. There may be short-term gains in pushing others around, but in the long run, power leads to unwilling cooperation rather than mutually beneficial relationships.

Whether manager or employee, you are likely to get more of what you want if you learn how to exercise influence rather than wield power. Sometimes confrontation is necessary, but is best resorted to after all else has been tried. Old-style managers and union leaders would do well to take note! Many of the examples of assertiveness versus aggressiveness on pages 160–62 apply to the workplace.

Rational Effectiveness Training at work

How RET can enhance the effectiveness of your workplace

The techniques of emotional control and behavioural change offered by Rational Effectiveness Training can benefit the workplace in two main ways. First, if people are able to control dysfunctional emotions, they will experience less distress and be free to use their emotional energy more productively. Second, RET can help people free up essential workplace skills that are often blocked by self-defeating thinking:

- *Conflict management* becomes more effective when the blocks to assertiveness are confronted.
- *Time management* is facilitated by dealing with avoidance and low frustration tolerance.
- *Communication skills* improve when managers and staff deal with the tension and low frustration tolerance that arise from beliefs such as: 'I must always look good in front of my colleagues', 'I must always receive the approval of my superiors', 'My subordinates must never think badly of me', and 'I should be able to communicate better.'
- *Delivery of performance appraisals* is facilitated when managers deal with the self-defeating beliefs that prevent them from providing accurate feedback to employees. Through RET they can learn to address their own high needs for approval, overconcern with negative

233

reactions from employees, and self-downing over their management performance.

- *Effective leadership* becomes a reality when managers develop flexible attitudes and an adaptive, change-oriented approach to new programmes and ideas.
- *Creative decision-making* becomes possible when internal blocks to change are addressed, especially self-defeating beliefs such as: 'We can't move ahead unless we are sure of success', 'Profits must always go up', 'I must always receive positive feedback from my superiors', and 'My employees must perceive me as a nice person.'

RET will improve performance — not lower it

Helping people learn new ways of dealing with their emotions and stress will, in the long run, increase their performance and effectiveness. Perfectionism, for example, paradoxically hinders excellence. Fears of failure or what others will think stops people from trying their hand at new things. High levels of anxiety slow people down and distract them from problem-solving. Hostility and resentment hinder effective teamwork.

Time put into Rational Effectiveness Training will be time well spent. It facilitates problem-solving and task-completion rather than avoidance and procrastination. It is aimed at helping people achieve excellence — and distress-free enjoyment.

The benefits RET can bring to the workplace are best summed up by listing how the Twelve Rational Principles can be applied to achieve effectiveness in that setting.

Applying the Twelve Rational Principles at work

Self-knowledge

- Know what you don't know. Acknowledging your shortcomings will keep you on the watch for new knowledge to improve your effectiveness.
- Know what you are suited to. A high-energy, risk- and stimulation-loving person will experience distress in a boring, repetitive job; alternatively, a low-energy, safety-conscious person will not cope well in a high-flying position.
- If you acknowledge your desires and weaknesses, you will be better able to maintain appropriate and safe boundaries in the workplace.

- Be clear about your limits. Be able to extend yourself, but know when to ease off to avoid any danger of burning out.

Self-acceptance and confidence

- If you accept yourself without self-rating, you will be able to take and use feedback — including constructive criticism — without feeling defensive.
- Confidence in specific abilities will enable you to use them to the maximum to achieve your goals and make yourself marketable to employers.
- Managers who do not need external evidence of their 'worth' will have less difficulty with the new participation model,[5] because they will not worry that it strips them of their power and authority.

Enlightened self-interest

- Make time to be supportive of others, then you will be supported in turn.
- Are you and your partner a two-career couple? Facilitating the other's career will make it more likely they will facilitate yours.
- If you are a manager, consultation and power-sharing will be in your interests in the long run. Help staff feel valued and in control of their work situation by being positive in your dealings with them. Emphasise what you want rather than what you don't. Exercise direct control only when there is no practicable alternative. Avoid reacting angrily, and handle complaints in a constructive manner. Give, and therefore invite, positive feedback. Acknowledge and reward special efforts. Helping your staff feel in control will keep you in control.

Tolerance for frustration and discomfort

- Accepting critical feedback on your performance is how you will learn and develop and hence increase your job satisfaction. View the discomfort this might bring as unpleasant but tolerable — and worth the gain.
- If you are a manager, accept the realities of your role. You *will* receive criticism from others. You *will* sometimes end up bearing responsibility for other peoples' mistakes. The smooth functioning of your

operation *will* be disrupted from time to time. If you consider such happenings as inevitable and uncomfortable, rather than intolerable and unbearable, you will be better able to take them in your stride.

Long-range enjoyment

- Rapid changes in the marketplace require a focus on the long term, and confident leadership able to resist pressure for short-term gains.
- Collective decision-making may take longer than simply making up your own mind and issuing an order, but it will save time in the long run when others, through being involved, make a genuine commitment to what is decided and see the job through.
- In the short run, you may prefer to be up to date with your paperwork; but taking time instead to support your coworkers could benefit you more in the long term.
- Confrontation may seem the quickest way to get what you want — and sometimes this will be the case — but winning people over with reasoning and friendliness will get you more in the long run.

Risk-taking

- Some businesses do go to the wall, but few would get off the ground in the first place if there was no-one with a vision prepared to take an initial step of faith.
- Choices will not always be black and white. Sometimes you will have to go with the best of the options open to you, without certainty of success. If you have trouble with this, check out the consequences of not making a decision.

Moderation

- To avoid burnout, beware of obsessiveness or overinvolvement with your work. Take regular breaks, especially when you feel a compulsion to keep on working. Go home when your colleagues do. Keep your work in balance with the rest of your life.
- Adopt a moderate approach to your dealings with coworkers and subordinates. Reasonableness and negotiation will create a less stressful environment than opinionatedness and obstinacy.
- Maintain appropriate boundaries. Be friendly, socialise and share

mutual support with coworkers or subordinates, but keep within limits that protect both you and them.

Emotional and behavioural responsibility

- Take responsibility for how you feel about your work and your responses to how you are treated. There may be dysfunctional elements to your workplace, but blaming others will just keep you a victim — and set you up for burnout.
- Emotional responsibility will reduce the time and energy workers and managers spend on self-defeating reactions to frustrating circumstances, and help them look for solutions.

Self-direction and commitment

- Workers are more likely to feel distress when they perceive a lack of power in respect of decisions that affect them, they have too much or too little work, there is under- or overpromotion, authority is not matched by responsibility, objectives or requirements are unclear, conflict exists between multiple job demands, or training is inadequate. Are you unsure what is expected of you in your job? If so, obtain clarification of what you are supposed to be achieving. If you lack the necessary training, ask for it or seek it out yourself. Decide what changes to your role you would like and negotiate on these.
- Self-directed people don't wait for things to happen or other people to do things to them. They see problems and initiate action and change. If they want support, they go and get it; in return, they watch out for colleagues who may be under stress and offer to lend a hand.
- Self-directed people do not feel a need to compete with their peers — they know what they want and work towards attaining it, without envying what others are achieving. Being non-competitive means having the freedom to enjoy mutually supportive relationships with colleagues.

Flexibility
Flexibility aids survival in organisations

- The modern workplace is characterised by significant changes in the composition of the workforce. There are, for example, increasing numbers of women and members of ethnic minorities, who bring to organisations new values, desires and goals. This requires companies to be flexible and adaptive, and free of rigid, absolutist attitudes that interfere with cooperation and problem-solving.

- There is a new level of major international competition. Businesses must be more alert than ever to changes in the marketplace and able to respond quickly, or even anticipate them.

- New technology means old methods are no longer satisfactory. Resistance to change can be costly. It can trigger distress for many people in an organisation, and sometimes even lead to organisational failure. Anticipating change rather than simply waiting for it to happen, as Bartol and Martin have pointed out, can significantly reduce any negative impact it may have.[6]

- Research has revealed that managers who do not cope well with stress fear change and tend to be inflexible and low in problem-solving ability. Those who cope better see organisational changes as challenges rather than threats, are flexible and adaptable, and are willing to try new ways of dealing with problems.[7] Effective supervisors, rather than dictating procedures which they ensure are rigidly applied, explain the aims of a job and provide guidelines for achieving these in a general fashion, leaving staff to accomplish the goals in their own way.[8]

Objective thinking

- The modern business setting is not a place for 'magical' thinking. It is necessary for commercial survival that feet be firmly on the ground. Make sure you are in touch with reality.

- Rid yourself especially of any myths about how human beings work. Study psychology. Know how to get the best out of people by appealing to their enlightened self-interest rather than moralising about what they 'should' do.

Acceptance of reality

- Be able to roll with the punches. No matter how well you do as an employee, as an executive, or as the boss, you are unlikely to succeed at everything to which you turn your hand. Acceptance of reality will help you avoid overreacting when things don't work out, and, instead of railing against fate, to pick yourself up and start again.

Further reading on effectiveness at work

Bramson, Robert M. *Coping with the Fast Track Blues*. Doubleday, New York, 1990.

Colbert, Audrey. *Dealing with Sexual Harassment: A New Zealand handbook for employers/employees, students and educators.* GP Books, Wellington, 1989.

Cuozzo, Jane Hershey, and Graham, S. Diane. *Side by Side Strategies: How two-career couples can thrive in the nineties.* Mastermedia Limited, New York, 1990.

Ellis, Albert. *Executive Leadership: A rational approach.* Institute for Rational Living, New York, 1972.

Hilsgen, Laurie, and Vause, Helen. *Working from Home in New Zealand.* GP Publications Ltd, Wellington, 1993.

Ingham, Christine. *Life Without Work: A time for change, growth and personal transformation.* HarperCollins Publishers, London, 1994.

Notes

Chapter 1
1. Selye, Hans. *Stress Without Distress*. Hodder & Stoughton, London, 1974.
2. Ibid.

Chapter 2
1. American Psychiatric Association. *Diagnostic and Statistical Manual of Mental Disorders,* 4th edn. Washington, DC, 1994.

Chapter 4
1. Cloninger, C.R., et al. 'A Psychobiological Model of Temperament and Character'. *Archives of General Psychiatry*, 50, 975–990, 1993; and Gregson, Olga, and Looker, Terry. 'The Biological Basis of Stress Management'. *British Journal of Guidance and Counselling*, 22:1, 13–26, 1994.
2. Bernard, Michael E. *Staying Rational in an Irrational World: Albert Ellis and Rational-Emotive Therapy*, p. 50. Lyle Stuart, New York, 1986.
3. Gregson and Looker, op. cit.
4. See Peele, Stanton, and DeGrandpre, Richard. 'My Genes Made Me Do It'. *Psychology Today*, 28:4, 50, 1995.
5. Booth-Kewley, S., and Friedman, H.S. 'Psychological Predictors of Heart Disease: A Quantitative Review'. *Psychological Bulletin*, 101, 343–62, 1987.
6. Rotter, Julian. 'Generalized Expectancies for Internal Versus External Control of Reinforcement'. *Psychological Monographs*, 80:1 (whole no. 609), 1966.
7. Asbell, Bernard. *What They Know About You*. Random House, New York, 1991.
8. Ellis, A., et al. *Rational-Emotive Therapy with Alcoholics and Substance Abusers.*

Allyn and Bacon, Boston, 1988.

Chapter 6
1. Burns, David. 'The Perfectionist's Script for Self-Defeat'. *Psychology Today* (Nov), 34–52, 1980.

Chapter 7
1. Cherry, Laurence. 'On The Real Benefits of Eustress: Interview with Hans Selye'. *Psychology Today* (Mar), 60–70, 1978.
2. Hauck, P.A. *Overcoming the Rating Game: Beyond Self-love — Beyond Self-esteem*. Westminster/John Knox, Louisville, KY, 1992.
3. Seligman, Martin E.P. *What You Can Change and What You Can't: The complete guide to successful self-improvement*. Random House, Sydney, 1994.
4. Cherry, op. cit.
5. Carroll, Lewis. *Through the Looking-glass (and What Alice Found There)*. 1872.
6. Kobasa, Suzanne C. 'Stressful Life Events, Personality, and Health: An Inquiry into Hardiness'. *Journal of Personality and Social Psychology*, 37:1, 1–11, 1979.
7. Reported in Asbell, Bernard. *What They Know About You*, p. 261. Random House, New York, 1991.
8. Kobasa, op. cit.
9. Von Oech, Roger. *A Whack on the Side of the Head*. Angus & Robertson Publishers, Sydney, 1984.
10. Burns, David. *Feeling Good: The new mood therapy*. Signet, New American Library, New York, 1980.
11. Seligman, op. cit.

12. A saying originally coined by a Taoist monk, popularised by Reinhold Niebuhr, adopted by Alcoholics Anonymous, paraphrased by Gunars Neiders in *The Conquest of Happiness: A rational approach* (found on the Internet at http://www.halcyon.com/neiders/conquest/conquest.htm), and further paraphrased by this author.

Chapter 8

1. DiMattia, Dominic, and Ijzermans, Theo. *Reaching Their Minds: A trainer's manual for Rational Effectiveness Training.* Institute for Rational-Emotive Therapy, New York, 1996.

2. Froggatt, Wayne. *Choose to Be Happy: Your step-by-step guide.* HarperCollins Publishers, Auckland, 1993.

3. A good selection of tapes is obtainable from the Albert Ellis Institute, 45 East 65th Street, New York 10021-6593, United States of America, fax 00-1-212-249-3582, phone 00-1-212-535-0822, Internet: http://www.iret.org/

Chapter 10

1. US Department of Health and Human Services. *Dietary Guidelines for Americans.* Washington, 1995.

2. King, Olwyn. *Good For You: The latest word on what to eat.* Dietwise Publications, Petone, New Zealand, 1993.

Chapter 11

1. Goldfried, M.R., and Davison, G.C. *Clinical Behaviour Therapy.* Holt, Rinehart and Winston, New York, 1976.

Chapter 12

1. Morin, C.M., et al. 'Cognitive-Behavior Therapy for Late-Life Insomnia'. *Journal of Consulting & Clinical Psychology*, 61:1, 137–46, 1993.

Chapter 13

1. Schultz, Duane P., & Schultz, Sydney E. *Psychology and Industry Today.* MacMillan Publishing Company, New York, 1990.

Chapter 14

1. Robb, Harold B. 'Why You Don't Have a "Perfect Right" to Anything'. *Journal of Rational-Emotive & Cognitive-Behavior Therapy*, 10:4, 259–70, 1992.

Chapter 16

1. Lakein, Alan. *How to Get Control of Your Time and Your Life.* Signet, New York, 1973.

2. The 80/20 rule — also known as the Pareto Principle — was developed by economist Vilfredo Pareto.

3. For material on 'time-extension' see: Levinson, Jay Conrad. *The 90-Minute Hour.* Penguin Books, New York, 1990.

4. See: Frank, Milo. *How to Run a Successful Meeting in Half the Time.* Simon and Schuster, New York, 1989.

5. Schlenger, Sunny, and Roesch, Roberta. *How to be Organized in Spite of Yourself.* Signet, New York, 1989.

Chapter 17

1. Cash, Grady. *Conquer the Seven Deadly Money Mistakes.* Center for Financial Well-Being, Rancho Cordova, CA (Internet — http://www.ns.net/cash/), 1994

Chapter 18

1. Asimov, Isaac. 'My Own View', in Holdstock, Robert T. (ed.). *The Encyclopedia of Science Fiction.* 1978.

2. Found on the Internet at http:/www.igs.net~mascot/quote.htm

3. Toffler, Alvin. *Future Shock.* Pan Books, London, 1970.

4. Holmes, T.H., and Rahe, R.H. 'The Social Readjustment Rating Scale'. *Jour-*

Notes

nal of Psychosomatic Research, 11, 213, 1967.

5. Toffler, Alvin. *Powershift: Knowledge, Wealth, and Violence at the Edge of the 21st Century.* Bantam Books, New York, 1990.

6. Sheehy, Gail. *New Passages: Mapping your life across time.* HarperCollins Publishers, London, 1996.

7. Toffler, op. cit., 1970.

8. Imber-Black, Evan, and Roberts, Janine. *Rituals for our Times.* Harper Perennial, New York, 1992.

Chapter 19

1. Froggatt, op. cit.

2. Maslow, A.H. *Motivation and Personality.* Harper & Row, New York, 1954.

Chapter 20

1. Palmer, Stephen, and Szymanska, Kasia. 'A Checklist for Clients Interested in Receiving Counselling, Psychotherapy or Hypnosis'. *The Rational Emotive Behaviour Therapist*, 2:1, 28–31, 1994.

Chapter 21

1. Freudenberger, H.J. *Burnout: The high cost of achievement.* Doubleday, New York, 1980.

2. Loftus, Mary. 'Frisky Business: Love at work'. *Psychology Today*, 28:2 (Mar–Apr), 34–85, 1995.

3. Schmidt, Stuart M., and Kipnis, David. 'The Perils of Persistence'. *Psychology Today* (Nov), 32–4, 1987.

4. Zuker, Elaina. *The Seven Secrets of Influence.* McGraw-Hill, Inc., New York, 1991.

5. Schultz, D.P., and Schultz, S.E. *Psychology and Industry Today.* Macmillan, New York, 1990.

6. Bartol, Kathryn M., and Martin, David C. *Management.* McGraw-Hill, New York, 1991.

7. Summers, L.S. 'Stress Management in Business Organizations'. *The Industrial-Organizational Psychologist*, 20:3, 29–33, 1983.

8. Sartain, A.Q., and Baker, A.W. *The Supervisor and the Job.* McGraw-Hill, New York, 1978.

Bibliography
Stress-Management Resources on the Internet

What follows is a list of resources relating to stress management which were on the Internet at the time this book was written. If you cannot connect to a particular site that is listed here, the server may be down or overloaded, so try again another day. However, because the Internet is constantly changing, the address may have changed or no longer exist. See if you can find it using one of the Internet search engines, such as Alta Vista. A search engine will also help you locate new resources for the topic you are investigating.

If you do not have a computer and Internet connection of your own, it is most likely your local library will be connected. You can probably use one of its computer terminals for a small hourly fee, and print out the information you want and take it with you.

Causes of stress
Bases of human behaviour — http://psych.lmu.edu/ahbe.htm
Moral development in humans — http://www.clark.net/pub/wright/introduc.htm
Values development — http://members.aol.com/evolvalues/index.html

Thinking and stress
Common unrealistic beliefs — http://www.cyberpsych.com/unreal_beliefs.html
How to avoid being gored by unicorns — http://prop1.org/park/unicorn.htm
The 'no nonsense' personality inventory — http://www.cyberpsych.com/nnpi.html
The exchange vocabulary — http://www.cyberpsych.com/vocab.html
Twelve irrational ideas — http://www.iret.org/essays/teorebta.html

The Twelve Rational Principles
Self-knowledge
Psychology tutorial — http://www.mindtools.com/page1swc.html
Personality tests — http://www1.usa1.com/~aycrumba/personality.html

Self-acceptance and confidence
Psychotherapy and the value of a human — http://www.iret.org/essays/value1.html
Showing people they are not worthless individuals — http://www.iret.org/essays/worth.html

Bibliography

Enlightened self-interest
Rational self-interest — http://calvin.linfield.edu/~dbrewer/self-int.html
Self- and social-interest exercise — http://www.clark.net/pub/sherman/self interest.html

Tolerance for frustration and discomfort
Discomfort and procrastination — http://www.iret.org/essays/procrst1.html
Discomfort and habit-resisting — http://rampages.onramp.net/~sarm/urges.html

Long-range enjoyment
Discussion of hedonism – http://www.geocities.com/Athens/Acropolis/2743/index.html

Risk-taking
Risk-taking and success — http://www.achievement.org/autodoc/atv/atv15stu–1

Moderation
Moderation and health — http://www.gartland.com/phoenix/95–6/6-guide.html
Harm reduction — http://www2.cac.washington.edu:1180/alumni/columns/march96/harms_way.html
Moderation and religion — http://student.uq.edu.au/~py101663/general/unhealth.htm

Emotional and behavioural responsibility
Responsibility Deficit Disorder — http://www.cmhc.com/perspectives/articles/art11964.htm
The no-cop-out therapy — http://www.iret.org/essays/tncot1.html

Self-direction and commitment
Self-direction and learning 1 — http://www.famu.edu/sjmga/ggrow/SSDL/MotivateNote.html
Self-direction and learning 2 — http://www.ncrel.org/sdrs/areas/issues/students/learning/lr200.htm
Self-direction and work — http://choo.fis.utoronto.ca/FIS/Courses/LIS1230/LIS1230sharma/motive2.htm

Flexibility
Change management — http://www.webcom.com/hrtmath/IHM/HMNL0502/Surfing.html
Flexibility and family rules — http://www.bradshawdifference.com/family.html

Bibliography

Flexibility at work — http://www.hslib.washington.edu/your_health/hbeat/hb950228.html
Flexibility, change and organisations — http://www.webcom.com/hrtmath/IHM/Articles/changemgt.html

Objective thinking
An introduction to logic — http://www.uoguelph.ca/~bmyers/logic.html
Brief introduction to the scientific method — http://www.indiana.edu/~gasser/science.html
Flexibility and the scientific method — http://village.ios.com/~rkc1/bridgman.shtml
Logic and the paranormal — http://www.csicop.org/si/9601/logic.html
Process of the scientific method — http://www.clc.uc.edu/~ladybug/bioclass/sci_meth.htmlx
Science and superstition — http://harpo.tnstate.edu/~folklore/vsuper.htm
The essence of Rational Emotive Behaviour Therapy — http://www.iret.org/essays/teorebta.html

Acceptance of reality
Acceptance of death — http://www.wwdc.com/death/creativity.html
Acceptance of pain — http://www.forthrt.com/~chronicl/archjune/musings.htm
Acknowledgement of reality — http://www.infi.net/~susanf/accept.htm
From denial to acceptance — http://www.usa.net/~ague/autism.html

Rational Effectiveness Training
Catalogue of tapes and self-help literature — http://www.iret.org/catalog.html
Homework assignments in psychotherapy — http://www.cyberpsych.com/homework.html
Stress diary — http://www.mindtools.com/smstrdia.html

Goal-setting
Personal goal-setting and time-management — http://www.mindtools.com
LifePlan (shareware for setting goals) — http://www.mindtools.com/lifeplan.html
Group goal-setting — http://www.open.org/scserv/i2goals.html
Family goal-setting — http://www.ag.ohio-state.edu/~ohioline/hyg-fact/5000/5211.html
Clarifying values — http://www.careersonline.com.au/disc/values.html
Choosing a career — http://www.careersonline.com.au/menu.html

Healthy living
Virtual Nutrition Centre — http://www-sci.lib.uci.edu/HSG/Nutrition.html
Human nutrition information files — http://leviathan.tamu.edu:70/pubs/humnutr/

Bibliography

Healthy.Net — *Nutrition Information Center* — http://www.healthy.net/nutrit/
Mind Tools on nutrition and exercise — http://www.mindtools.com/smhealth.html
Keeping Healthy (exercise information sheet) — http://www.mcchiro.com/keeping.htm
American Psychological Association on exercise and stress — http://helping.apa.org/neurala.html
Exercise and stress reduction — http://www.familyinternet.com/mhc/top/002081.htm

Relaxation
Relaxation, imagery, breath control — http://www.mindtools.com/smpmr.html
Breathing — http://cybertowers.com/selfhelp/articles/stress/breath.html
Breathing (alternative view) — http://cybertowers.com/selfhelp/articles/health/relax.html
Meditation and relaxation — http://www.healthy.net/library/articles/DanRedwood/meditat.htm
Relaxation for surgical patients — http://198.185.157.25/ajn/5.5/a505038e.1t
Diaphragmatic breathing — http://www.algy.com/anxiety/diaph.html
Biofeedback — http://www.primenet.com/~thielbl/
Obtaining a relaxation tape: A professionally prepared recording of the three-stage relaxation method, with the breathing-focus technique included, is available for purchase. The best way to obtain this cassette tape and instruction booklet package is to use the Internet — http://www.voyager.co.nz/~rational/public/resources.htm

Sleep problems
National Sleep Foundation on sleep disorders — http://www.iacnet.com/health/15033666.htm
Sleep disorders test — http://nshsleep.com/howwell.html
The sleep medicine home page — http://www.cloud9.net/~thorpy/
The sleep better guide — http://www.sitnsleep.com/sleep/guide.html
Sleepnet list of resources — http://www.sleepnet.com/

Getting support
Addictive relationships — http://www.odos.uiuc.edu/Counseling_Center/addict.htm
Beliefs and loneliness — http://www.hci.net/~waynew/WRBrassell/wbrassell_thoughts.html
Communication and health — http://www.uiuc.edu/departments/mckinley/health-info/hlthpro/relation/communic.html
Couples communication — http://www.iret.org/essays/hntgyah1.html

Bibliography

Friendship evaluation test — http://www.hci.net/~waynew/WRBrassell/wbrassell_test2.html

Friendship qualities test — http://www.uiuc.edu/departments/mckinley/health-info/hlthpro/relation/qualfrnd.html

Intimate relationships — http://www.stresscure.com/relation/succeed.html

Isolation test — http://www.hci.net/~waynew/WRBrassell/wbrassell_test1.html

Listening skills — http://www.stresscure.com/relation/7keys.html

Loneliness support — http://point-2-point.com/ssl/index.html

Making friends — http://www.uiuc.edu/departments/mckinley/health-info/hlthpro/relation/friends.html

Marital problems — http://www.iret.org/essays/tnodmil.html

Non-verbal communication test — http://zzyx.ucsc.edu/~archer/

Obstacles to friendship — http://www.hci.net/~waynew/WRBrassell/wbrassell_obstacles.html

Online support groups — http://www.support-group.com/faq.htm#supportlinks

Relationship suggestions survey — http://newciv.org/worldtrans/BOV/relationships.html

Shyness — http://www.uiuc.edu/departments/mckinley/health-info/hlthpro/relation/shyness.html

Shyness reading list — http://www.shyness.com/shyness-reading-list.html

Singles, dating and relationships — http://www.successways.com/

Social-mindedness test — http://www.uiuc.edu/departments/mckinley/health-info/hlthpro/relation/socially.html

Stress in relationships — http://www.stresscure.com/14dycure/chapt10.html

Verbal and non-verbal communication — http://www.mixteca.com/relating/ch9.html

Assertiveness

Aggression — http://www.iret.org/essays/aggress1.html

Assertiveness quiz — http://theoaktree.com/assrtquz.htm

Assertiveness quiz 2 — http://www.queendom.com/assert.html

Assertiveness self-test — http://www.putnam.com/putnam/books/psych_book_self_tests/excerpt.html

Assertiveness tip sheet — http://www.tufts.edu/hr/test/tips/assert.html

Assertiveness, aggressiveness, unassertiveness — http://gossamer.saf.uwplatt.edu/counsel/esteem/assertvs.htm

Medication and assertiveness — http://newciv.org/worldtrans/GIB/reinv/RIS–81.HTML

Parental assertiveness — http://rainbow.rmi.net/~ddow/tlisci.html

Sexual assertiveness — http://207.123.208.13/life/health/sexualit/behave/lhsbe002.htm

Unassertive response styles — http://www.swin.edu.au/hr/staff-dev/assert3.htm

Bibliography

Active living

Active living — http://www.activeliving.ca/activeliving/go4green/provinces/ab/alvol153.html

Active living for families — http://www.gov.ab.ca./~mcd/arl/rec/recfacts/100/fax146.htm

Activity and ageing — http://www.gov.ab.ca./~mcd/arl/rec/recfacts/100/fax129.htm

Listing of Internet hobby/craft sites — http://africa.cis.co.za/ent/recr3.html

Motivating children to be active — http://www.gov.ab.ca./~mcd/arl/rec/recfacts/100/fax103.htm

Motivation for activity — http://www.gov.ab.ca./~mcd/arl/rec/recfacts/100/fax106.htm

Physical activity for people with disabilities — http://www.gov.ab.ca./~mcd/arl/rec/recfacts/100/fax130.htm

Recreation for older adults — http://www.gov.ab.ca./~mcd/arl/rec/recfacts/600/fax603.htm

Recreation in the workplace — http://www.gov.ab.ca./~mcd/arl/rec/recfacts/600/fax606.htm

Recreation in the workplace 2 — http://www.gov.ab.ca./~mcd/arl/rec/recfacts/600/fax607.htm

Recreational ideas listing — http://sfbay.yahoo.com/Sports_and_Recreation/

Time management

Dealing with time-wasters — http://www.smartbiz.com/sbs/arts/sap1.htm

Making time — http://ianrwww.unl.edu/ianr/pubs/nebfacts/nf94–173.htm

Mind Tools on time management — http://www.mindtools.com/page5.html

Overcoming procrastination — http://www.iret.org/essays/procrst1.html

References on procrastination — http://www.cs.ucla.edu/~pierce/procrastination.html

Time management at home — http://ianrwww.unl.edu/ianr/pubs/nebfacts/nf94–174.htm

Time management for children — http://www.pace-ed.com/homenews.html

Time management for couples — http://www.herspace.com/herspace/other/timemanagement.html

Time management for students — http://www.d.umn.edu/student/loon/acad/strat/time_man_princ.html

Time management myths — http://www.oswego.edu/~baldwin/Time-Management.html

Time use log and audit — http://www.d.umn.edu/student/loon/acad/strat/time_audit.html

Work habits and time management — http://classes.ag.uiuc.edu/FSHN350/timemgmt.html

Bibliography

Managing financial and material resources

Buying smart — http://www.pueblo.gsa.gov/1997crh/res_prt1.txt
Center for Financial Well-Being — http://www.ns.net/cash/
Debt management library — http://members.aol.com/debtrelief/Library.html
Electronic credit repair kit — http://www.primenet.com/~kielsky/credit.html
FinanCenter — http://www.financenter.com/
Free stuff — http://home.earthlink.net/~boughter/Assorted.html
Frugal Corner — http://www.best.com/~piner/frugal.html
Getting your budget to balance — http://www.stretcher.com/stories/970113b.htm
Money matters for young adults — ttp://members.aol.com/greenzine/whatsgrn.html
Recovery from debt — http://www.voicenet.com/~blowry/debt.html
Retirement planning — http://tours.excite.com/go.webx?128@^68920@.ee6bcd9/0
Solving money problems — http://www.icis.on.ca/homepages/ccslondon/ccl.htm
The Cheapskate Monthly — http://www.cheapsk8.com/
The Dollar Stretcher — http://www.stretcher.com/dollar/

Managing change

Alvin Toffler on change — http://www.physics.wisc.edu/~shalizi/New ScientistArticles/alvin-toffler/
Attitudes to change — http://www.mindtools.com/smchange.html
Resistance to change — http://www.catch22.com/lln/s_faq.html#resistant
Stress and change — http://www.catch22.com/lln/s_main.html
Surviving organisational change — http://www.stresscure.com/jobstress/reorg.html
The Social Readjustment Rating Scale — http://www.webcast1.com/icp/stresste.htm

Problem-solving

A real life application: Problem solving after a divorce — http://www.divorcehelp.com/SC/C42Structured.html
Brainstorming 1 — http://anime.tcp.com/~prime8/Orbit/Brainstorm/index.html
Brainstorming 2 — http://www.mindtools.com/brainstm.html
Decision trees — http://www.mindtools.com/dectree.html
Mind Mapping — http://www.mindman.com/
PMI approach to decision-making — http://www.mindtools.com/pmi.html
Skills for locating information — http://www.lib.utc.edu/bigsix.html
Workplace problem-solving — http://www.all-biz.com/problem.htm

Seeking help
Using counselling and psychotherapy

Choosing a psychologist — http://www.apa.org/pubinfo/howto.html
Choosing a therapist — http://abulafia.st.hmc.edu/~mmiles/faq.html

Bibliography

Introduction to cognitive-behaviour therapy — http://pages.nyu.edu/~lqh6007/BehavioralAssociates/index.html
Making an informed choice — http://www.therapist-list.com/infochoi.htm
Psychologist's code of conduct — http://www.apa.org/ethics/code.html
Questions about counsellors and psychotherapists — http://www.counselorlink.com/
Rate your psychotherapist — http://www.cybercouch.com/library/rati.tag.html
The essence of Rational Emotive Behaviour Therapy — http://www.iret.org/essays/teorebta.html
The no-cop-out therapy — http://www.iret.org/essays/tncot1.html
Types of therapists — http://members.aol.com/therapy678/freud/choice.htm

Tools for self-help
Albert Ellis Institute — http://www.iret.org/essays/
CyberCouch — http://www.cybercouch.com/
CyberPsychologist — http://www.cyberpsych.com/althome.html
Internet mental health — http://www.mentalhealth.com/p.html
Lay person's guide to psychotherapeutic medication — http://www.onlinepsych.com/treat/drugs.htm#N3
Mental Health Net self-help resources — http://www.cmhc.com/selfhelp.htm
Mind Tools — http://www.mindtools.com/
Psychology for living — http://www.gov.nb.ca/hotlist/psychology.htm
Rational Recovery — http://www.rational.org/recovery/
Self-help and Psychology *magazine* — http://cybertowers.com/selfhelp/articles/index.html
SMART Recovery — http://www.cybersych.com/smart.html

Workplace effectiveness
Rational Effectiveness Training — http://www.iret.org/essays/train1.html
Management psychology — http://www.mindtools.com/page10.html
Leadership skills — http://www.mindtools.com/page13.html
New styles of leadership — ttp://www.businessjournals.com/fcbj/fcbj_0403/jones.html
Choosing a new career — http://www.inst-mgt.org.uk/institute/support/career/adv_g2.html
Personal Development Planning Checklist — http://www.inst-mgt.org.uk/institute/support/chk–92.html
Management theory — http://unccvm.uncc.edu/~kecurran/lect–02.htm

General
These sites are especially relevant for general information on rational approaches to stress management and Rational Effectiveness Training.

Rational Training Programs (the author's web-site) — http://www.voyager.co.nz/
~train/
New Zealand Centre for Rational Emotive Behaviour Therapy — http://www.
voyager.co.nz/~rational/
Albert Ellis Institute (New York) — http://www.iret.org/
CyberPsychologist — http://www.cyberpsych.com/

Professional Books and Articles on Stress Management

The causes of stress

Gribbin, John, and Gribben, Mary. *Being Human: Putting people in an evolutionary perspective.* J M Dent, London, 1993.
Palmer, Stephen. *Stress Management: A course reader.* Centre for Stress Management, London, 1992.
Toates, F. *Biological Foundations of Behaviour.* Open University, Milton Keynes, 1988.

Thinking and stress

DiGiuseppe, Raymond. 'The Nature of Irrational and Rational Beliefs: Progress in Rational Emotive Behaviour Therapy'. *Journal of Rational-Emotive and Cognitive-Behaviour Therapy*, 14:1, 5–28, 1996.
Himle, David P. 'Changing Personal Rules'. *Journal of Rational-Emotive and Cognitive-Behaviour Therapy*, 7:2, 79–92, 1989.
Ruth, William J. 'Irrational Thinking in Humans: An evolutionary proposal for Ellis' genetic postulate'. *Journal of Rational-Emotive and Cognitive-Behaviour Therapy*, 10:1, 3–20, 1992.

Low discomfort/frustration tolerance

Ellis, Albert. 'A Sadly Neglected Cognitive Element in Depression'. *Cognitive Therapy and Research*, 11, 121–46, 1987.
Ellis, Albert. 'Discomfort Anxiety: A New Cognitive Behavioral Construct'. In Ellis, A., and Greiger, R. (eds). *Handbook of Rational-Emotive Therapy*, vol. 2. Springer, New York, 1986.

Rational Effectiveness Training

Cayer, M., et al. 'Conquering Evaluation Fear'. *Personnel Administrator*, 33:6, 97–107, 1988.

Bibliography

DiMattia, D., and Yeager, R. *Emotional Management: A necessary ingredient in corporate training and development workshops*. Institute for Rational-Emotive Therapy, New York, 1987.

DiMattia, D. 'A "Fast Track" Counselling Approach for EAPs'. *Benefits Today* (Nov), 1986.

DiMattia, D., et al. 'Emotional Barriers to Learning'. *Personnel Journal*, 68:11, 86–9, 1989.

DiMattia, Dominic, and Ijzermans, Theo. *Reaching Their Minds: A trainer's manual for rational effectiveness training*. Institute for Rational-Emotive Therapy, New York, 1996.

Dryden, Windy. *Creativity in Rational-Emotive Therapy*. Gale Centre Publications, Loughton, Essex, 1990.

Ellis, Albert, and DiMattia, Dominic. *Rational Effectiveness Training: A new method of facilitating management and labor relations*. Institute for Rational-Emotive Therapy, New York, 1991.

Forman, S.G., and Forman, B.D. 'Rational-Emotive Staff Development'. *Psychology in the Schools*, 17, 90–96, 1980.

Klarreich, S.H., et al. 'EAPs: Mind Over Myths'. *Personnel Administrator*, 32:2, 119–21, 1987.

Neenan, Michael. 'Rational-Emotive Therapy at Work'. *Stress News*, 5:1, 7–10, 1993.

Palmer, S. and Dryden, W. 'A Multimodal Approach to Stress Management'. *Stress News*, 3:1, 2–10, 1991.

Richman, D.R. (guest ed.). 'Working Together: Belief systems of individuals and organisations'. *Journal of Cognitive Psychotherapy*, 6:4, 231–44, 1992.

Walen, Susan R., et al. *A Practitioner's Guide to Rational-Emotive Therapy*, 2nd edn. Oxford, New York, 1992.

Watson, Julie. 'Good Race Relations in the Workplace'. *Mental Health News* (Mental Health Foundation of New Zealand) (Sep), p. 10, 1996.

Healthy living

Egger, Gary, and Swinburn, Boyd. *The Fat Loss Handbook: A guide for professionals*. Allen & Unwin, Sydney, 1996.

Goleman, Daniel, and Gurin, Joel (eds). *Mind/Body Medicine*. Consumer Reports Books, New York, 1993.

Relaxation training

Goldfried, M.R., and Davison, G.C. *Clinical Behaviour Therapy*. Holt, Rinehart & Winston, New York, 1976.

Palmer, Stephen. *Stress Management: A course reader*. Centre for Stress Management, London, 1992.

Sleep problems

Morin C.M., et al. 'Cognitive-Behavior Therapy for Late-Life Insomnia'. *Journal of Consulting and Clinical Psychology*, 61:1, 137–46, 1993.

Sloan E.P., et al. 'The Nuts and Bolts of Behavioral Therapy for Insomnia'. *Journal of Psychosomatic Research*, 37, supp. 1, 19–37, 1993.

Assertiveness

Carmody, T.P. 'Rational-Emotive, Self-Instructional, and Behavioral Assertion Training: Facilitation Maintenance'. *Cognitive Therapy and Research*, 2, 241–53, 1978.

Lange, A., and Jakubowski, P. *Responsible Assertive Behaviour: Cognitive-behavioural procedures for trainers.* Research Press, Champaign, Ill., 1976.

Robb, Harold B. 'Why You Don't Have a "Perfect Right" to Anything'. *Journal of Rational-Emotive and Cognitive-Behavior Therapy*, 10:4, 259–69, 1992.

Wolfe, J.L., and Fodor, I.G. 'A Cognitive-Behavioral Approach to Modifying Assertive Behavior in Women'. *Counselling Psychologist*, 5:4, 45–52, 1975.

Managing change

Palmer, Stephen. *Stress Management: A course reader.* Centre for Stress Management, London, 1992.

Seeking help

Palmer, Stephen, and Szymanska, Kasia. 'A Checklist for Clients Interested in Receiving Counselling, Psychotherapy or Hypnosis'. *The Rational Emotive Behaviour Therapist*, 2:1, 25–7, 1994.

Workplace effectiveness

See listing under 'Rational Effectiveness Training'.

Index

Index

Index